Mouth-Watering Mediterranean Recipes for Lunch & Dinner

Make Your Every Meal A Mediterranean Meal

By
Delia Bell

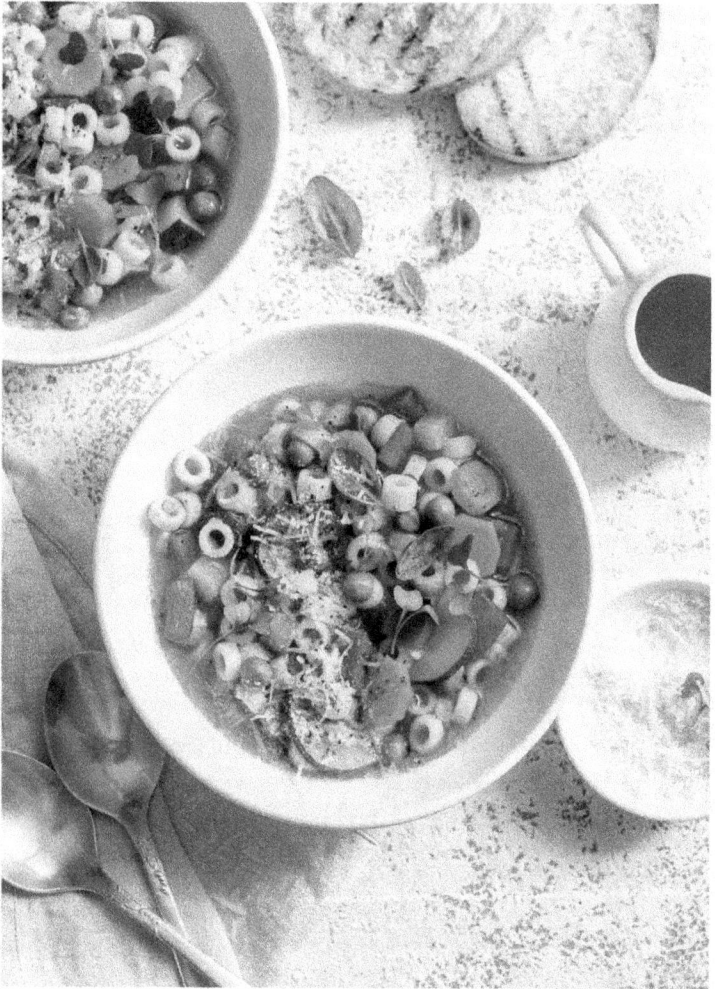

as such, any inattention, use, or misuse of the information in question by the reader will render any resulting actions solely under their purview. There are no scenarios in which the publisher or the original author of this work can be in any fashion deemed liable for any hardship or damages that may befall them after undertaking information described herein.

Additionally, the information in the following pages is intended only for informational purposes and should thus be thought of as universal. As befitting its nature, it is presented without assurance regarding its prolonged validity or interim quality. Trademarks that are mentioned are done without written consent and can in no way be considered an endorsement from the trademark holder.

Table of Contents

INTRODUCTION

What is the Mediterranean Diet?

The Mediterranean diet is based on the diets of traditional eating habits from the 1960s of people from countries that surround the Mediterranean Sea, such as Greece, Italy, and Spain, and it encourages the consumption of fresh, seasonal, and local foods. The Mediterranean diet has become popular because individuals show low rates of heart disease, chronic disease, and obesity. The Mediterranean diet profile focuses on whole grains, good fats (fish, olive oil, nuts etc.), vegetables, fruits, fish, and very low consumption of any non-fish meat. Along with food, the Mediterranean diet emphasizes the need to spend time eating with family and physical activity. The Mediterranean diet is not a single prescribed diet, but rather a general food-based eating pattern, which is marked by local and cultural differences throughout the Mediterranean region.

The diet is generally characterized by a high intake of plant-based foods (e.g. fresh fruit and vegetables, nuts, and cereals) and olive oil, a moderate intake of fish and poultry, and low intakes of dairy products (mostly yoghurt and cheese), red and processed meats, and sweets. Wine is typically consumed in moderation and, normally, with a meal. A strong focus is placed on social and cultural aspects, such as communal mealtimes, resting after eating, and regular physical activity. Nowadays, however, the diet is no longer followed as widely as it was 30-50 years ago, as the diets of people living in these regions are becoming more 'Westernized' and higher in energy dense foods.

Benefits
The Mediterranean diet is not a weight loss, but increasing fiber intake and cutting out red meat, animal fats, and processed food may lead to weight loss. People who follow the diet may also have a lower risk of various diseases.

Heart health
In the 1950s,an American scientist, found that people living in the poorer areas of southern Italy had a lower risk of heart disease and death than those in wealthier parts of New York. Dr. Keys attributed this to diet. Since then, many studies have indicated that following a Mediterranean diet can help the body maintain healthy cholesterol levels and reduce the risk of high blood pressure and cardiovascular disease. The overall pattern of the Mediterranean diet is similar to their own dietary recommendations. A high proportion of

calories on the diet come from fat, which can increase the risk of obesity. However, they also note that this fat is mainly unsaturated, which makes it a more healthful option than that from the typical American diet.

Protection from disease
The Mediterranean diet focuses on plant-based foods, and these are good sources of antioxidants.

The Mediterranean diet might offer protection from various cancers, and especially colorectal cancer. The reduction in risk may stem from the high intake of fruits, vegetables, and whole grains. By sticking to Mediterranean meals, people's levels of blood glucose and fats had decreased. During this time, there was also a lower incidence of stroke.

Diabetes
The Mediterranean diet may help prevent type 2 diabetes and improve markers of diabetes in people who already have the condition. Various other studies have concluded that following the Mediterranean diet can reduce the risk of type 2 diabetes and cardiovascular disease, which often occur together.

Food to eat
There is no single definition of the Mediterranean diet, but one group of scientists used the following as their

2015 basis of research.

Vegetables: Include 3 to 9 servings a day.

Fresh fruit: Up to 2 servings a day.

Cereals: Mostly whole grain from 1 to 13 servings a day.

Oil: Up to 8 servings of extra virgin (cold pressed) olive oil a day.

Fat — mostly unsaturated — made up 37% of the total calories. Unsaturated fat comes from plant sources, such as olives and avocado. The Mediterranean diet also provided 33 grams (g) of fiber a day. The baseline diet for this study provided around 2,200 calories a day. Typical ingredients. Here are some examples of ingredients that people often include in the Mediterranean diet.

Vegetables: Tomatoes, peppers, onions, eggplant, zucchini, cucumber, leafy green vegetables, plus others.

Fruits: Melon, apples, apricots, peaches, oranges, and lemons, and so on.

Legumes: Beans, lentils, and chickpeas.

Nuts and seeds: Almonds, walnuts, sunflower seeds, and cashews.

Unsaturated fat: Olive oil, sunflower oil, olives, and avocados.

Dairy products: Cheese and yogurt are the main dairy foods.

Cereals: These are mostly whole grain and include wheat and rice with bread accompanying many meals.

Fish: Sardines and other oily fish, as well as oysters and other shellfish. Poultry: Chicken or turkey.

Eggs: Chicken, quail, and duck eggs.

Drinks: A person can drink red wine in moderation.

The Mediterranean diet does not include strong liquor or carbonated and sweetened drinks. According to one definition, the diet limits red meat and sweets to less than 2 servings per week.

Food to avoid

Here's a list of foods you should generally limit while eating Mediterranean-style meals. Heavily processed foods. Let's be real: Many, many foods are processed to some degree. A can of beans has been processed, in the sense that the beans have been cooked before being canned. Olive oil has been processed, because olives have been turned into oil. But when we talk about limiting processed foods, this really means avoiding things like frozen meals with tons of sodium. You should also limit soda, desserts and candy. As the adage goes, if the ingredient list includes items that your great-grandparents wouldn't recognize as food, it's probably processed. If you're buying a packaged food that's as close to its whole-food form as possible — such as frozen fruit or veggies with nothing added — you're good to go.

Processed red meat

On the Mediterranean diet, you should minimize your intake of red meat, such as steak. What about processed red meat, such as hot dogs and bacon? You should avoid these foods or limit them as much as possible. A study published in BMJ found that regularly eating red meat, especially processed varieties, was associated with a higher risk of death. Butter. Here's another food that should be limited on the Mediterranean diet. Use olive oil instead, which has many heart health benefits and contains less saturated fat than butter. According to the USDA National Nutrient Database, butter has 7 grams of saturated fat per tablespoon, while olive oil has about 2 grams.

Refined grains

The Mediterranean diet is centered around whole grains, such as farro, millet, couscous and brown rice. With this eating style, you'll generally want to limit your intake of refined grains such as white pasta and white bread.

Alcohol

When you're following the Mediterranean diet, red wine should be your chosen alcoholic drink. This is because red wine offers health benefits, particularly for the heart. But it's important to limit intake of any type of alcohol to up to one drink per day for women, as well as men older than 65, and up to two drinks daily for men age 65 and younger. The amount that counts as a drink is 5 ounces of wine, 12 ounces of beer or 1.5 ounces of 80-proof liquor.

Creamy Salmon Soup

Servings: 6
Cooking Time: 15 Minutes

Ingredients:
- 2 tablespoon olive oil
- 1 red onion, chopped
- Salt and white pepper to the taste
- 3 gold potatoes, peeled and cubed
- 2 carrots, chopped
- 4 cups fish stock
- 4 ounces salmon fillets, boneless and cubed
- ½ cup heavy cream
- 1 tablespoon dill, chopped

Directions:
1. Heat up a pan with the oil over medium heat, add the onion, and sauté for 5 minutes.
2. Add the rest of the ingredients except the cream, salmon and the dill, bring to a simmer and cook for 5-6 minutes more.
3. Add the salmon, cream and the dill, simmer for 5 minutes more, divide into bowls and serve.

Nutrition Info: calories 214, fat 16.3, fiber 1.5, carbs 6.4, protein 11.8 112. Grilled Salmon With

Cucumber Dill Sauce

Servings: 4
Cooking Time: 40 Minutes

Ingredients:
- 4 salmon fillets
- 1 teaspoon smoked paprika
- 1 teaspoon dried sage
- Salt and pepper to taste
- 4 cucumbers, sliced
- 2 tablespoons chopped dill
- ½ cup Greek yogurt
- 1 tablespoon lemon juice
- 1 tablespoon olive oil

Directions:
1. Season the salmon with salt, pepper, paprika and sage.
2. Heat a grill pan over medium flame and place the salmon on the grill.
3. Cook on each side for 4 minutes.
4. For the sauce, mix the cucumbers, dill, yogurt, lemon juice and oil in a bowl. Add salt and pepper and mix well.
5. Serve the salmon with the cucumber sauce.

Nutrition Info: Per Serving:Calories:224 Fat:10.3g
Protein:26.3g Carbohydrates:8.9g

Grilled Basil-lemon Tofu Burgers

Servings: 6

Cooking Time: 6 Minutes

Ingredients:

- 6 slices (1/4-inch thick each) tomato
- 6 pieces (1 1/2-ounce) whole-wheat hamburger buns
- 1 pound tofu, firm or extra-firm, drained
- 1 cup watercress, trimmed
- Cooking spray
- 1/3 cup fresh basil, finely chopped
- 2 tablespoons Dijon mustard
- 2 tablespoons honey
- 1/4 cup freshly squeezed lemon juice
- 2 teaspoons grated lemon rind
- 1 tablespoon olive oil, extra-virgin,
- 1/2 teaspoon salt
- 1/4 teaspoon black pepper (freshly ground)
- 3 garlic cloves, minced
- 1 garlic cloves, minced
- 1/3 cup Kalamata olives, finely, chopped pitted
- 3 tablespoons sour cream, reduced-fat
- 3 tablespoons light mayonnaise

Directions:

1. Combine the marinade ingredients in a small-sized bowl. In a crosswise direction, cut the tofu into 6 slices. Pat each

piece dry using paper towels. Place them in a jelly roll pan and brush both sides of the slices with the marinade mixture; reserve any leftover marinade. Marinate for 1 hour.

2. Preheat the grill and coat the grill rack with cooking spray. Place the tofu slices; grill for about 3 minutes per side, brushing the tofu with the reserved marinade mixture.

3. In a small-sized bowl, combine the garlic-olive mayonnaise ingredients. Spread about 1 1/2 tablespoons of the mixture over the bottom half of the hamburger buns. Top each with 1 slice tofu, 1 slice tomato, about 2 tablespoons of watercress, and top with the top buns.

Nutrition Info:Per Serving:276 Cal, 11.3 g total fat (1.9 g sat. fat, 5.7 g mono fat, 2.2 g poly fat), 10.5 g protein, 34.5 g carb., 1.5 g fiber, 5 mg chol., 2.4 mg iron, 743 mg sodium, and 101 mg calcium.

Creamy Green Pea Pasta

Servings: 4

Cooking Time: 25 Minutes

Ingredients:

- 8 oz. whole wheat spaghetti
- 1 cup green peas
- 1 avocado, peeled and cubed
- 2 tablespoons olive oil
- 2 garlic cloves, chopped
- 2 mint leaves
- 1 tablespoon lemon juice
- ¼ cup heavy cream
- 2 tablespoons vegetable stock
- Salt and pepper to taste

Directions:

1. Pour a few cups of water in a deep pot and bring to a boil with a pinch of salt.

2. Add the spaghetti and cook for 8 minutes then drain well.

3. For the sauce, combine the remaining ingredients in a blender and pulse until smooth.

4. Mix the cooked spaghetti with the sauce and serve the pasta fresh.

Nutrition Info: Per Serving:Calories:294 Fat:20.1g Protein:6.4g Carbohydrates:25.9g

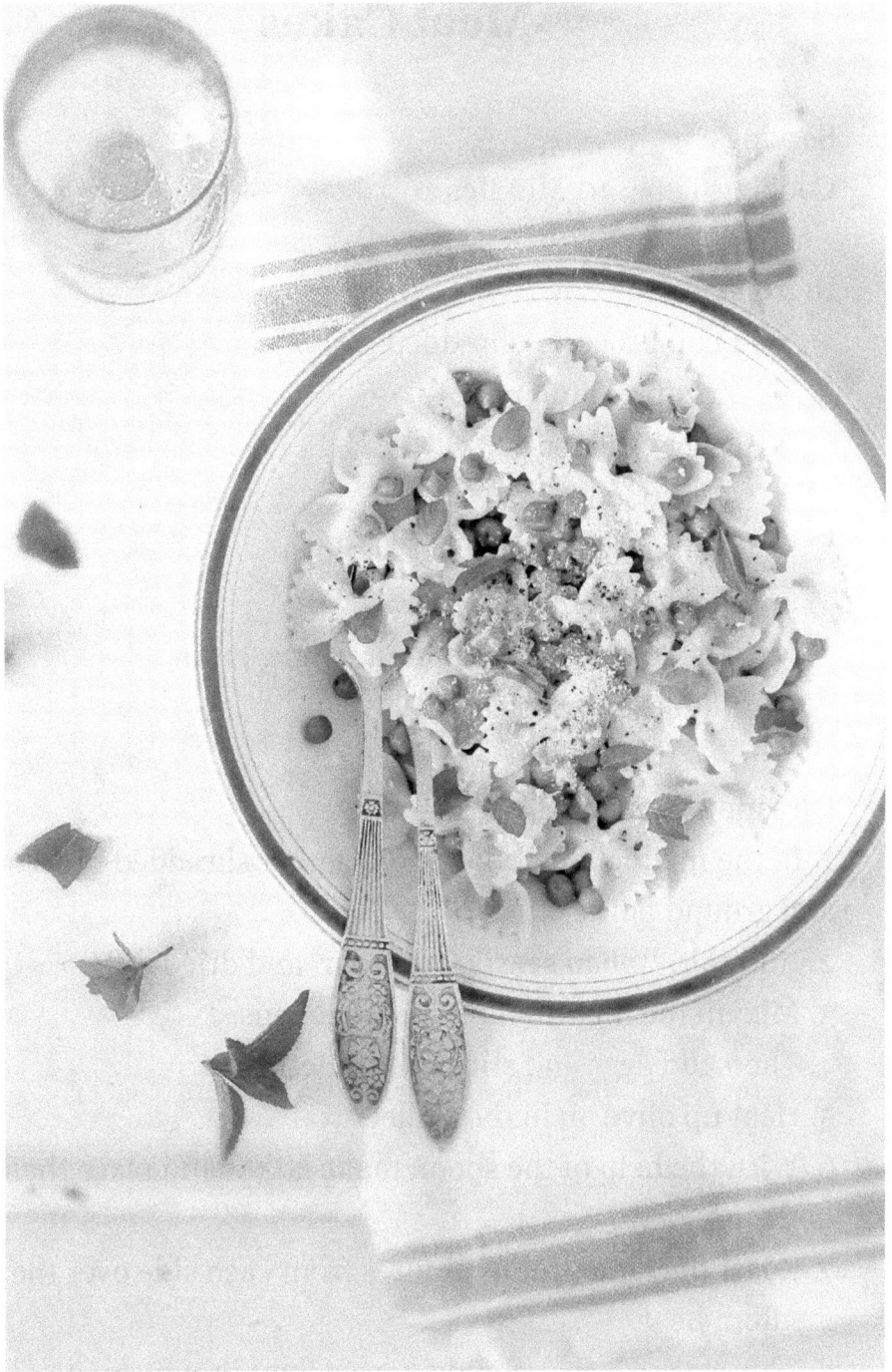

Meat Cakes

Servings: 4
Cooking Time: 10 Minutes

Ingredients:
- 1 cup broccoli, shredded
- ½ cup ground pork
- 2 eggs, beaten
- 1 teaspoon salt
- 1 tablespoon Italian seasonings
- 1 teaspoon olive oil
- 3 tablespoons wheat flour, whole grain
- 1 tablespoon dried dill

Directions:

1. In the mixing bowl combine together shredded broccoli and ground pork,

2. Add salt, Italian seasoning, flour, and dried dill.

3. Mix up the mixture until homogenous.

4. Then add eggs and stir until smooth.

5. Heat up olive oil in the skillet.

6. With the help of the spoon make latkes and place them in the hot oil.

7. Roast the latkes for 4 minutes from each side over the medium heat.

8. The cooked latkes should have a light brown crust.

9. Dry the latkes with the paper towels if needed.

Nutrition Info:Per Serving:calories 143, fat 6, fiber 0.9, carbs 7, protein 15.1

Herbed Roasted Cod

Servings: 4

Cooking Time: 45 Minutes

Ingredients:

- 4 cod fillets
- 4 parsley sprigs
- 2 cilantro sprigs
- 2 basil sprigs
- 1 lemon, sliced
- Salt and pepper to taste
- 2 tablespoons olive oil

Directions:

1. Season the cod with salt and pepper.

2. Place the parsley, cilantro, basil and lemon slices at the bottom of a deep dish baking pan.

3. Place the cod over the herbs and cook in the preheated oven at 350F for 15 minutes.

4. Serve the cod warm and fresh with your favorite side dish.

Nutrition Info: Per Serving:Calories:192 Fat:8.1g Protein:28.6g Carbohydrates:0.1g

Mushroom Soup

Servings: 2
Cooking Time: 20 Minutes

Ingredients:
- 1 cup cremini mushrooms, chopped
- 1 cup Cheddar cheese, shredded
- 2 cups of water
- ½ teaspoon salt
- 1 teaspoon dried thyme
- ½ teaspoon dried oregano
- 1 tablespoon fresh parsley, chopped
- 1 tablespoon olive oil
- 1 bell pepper, chopped

Directions:
1. Pour olive oil in the pan.
2. Add mushrooms and bell pepper. Roast the vegetables for 5 minutes over the medium heat.
3. Then sprinkle them with salt, thyme, and dried oregano.
4. Add parsley and water. Stir the soup well.
5. Cook the soup for 10 minutes.
6. After this, blend the soup until it is smooth and simmer it for 5 minutes more.
7. Add cheese and stir until cheese is melted.

8. Ladle the cooked soup into the bowls. It is recommended to serve soup hot.

Nutrition Info:Per Serving:calories 320, fat 26, fiber 1.4, carbs 7.4, protein 15.7

Salmon Parmesan Gratin

Servings: 4
Cooking Time: 45 Minutes

Ingredients:
- 4 salmon fillets, cubed
- 2 garlic cloves, chopped
- 1 fennel bulb, sliced
- ½ teaspoon ground coriander
- ½ teaspoon Dijon mustard
- ½ cup vegetable stock
- 1 cup heavy cream
- 2 eggs
- Salt and pepper to taste
- 1 cup grated Parmesan cheese

Directions:
1. Combine the salmon, garlic, fennel, coriander and mustard in a small deep dish baking pan.
2. Mix the eggs with cream and stock and pour the mixture over the fish.
3. Top with Parmesan cheese and bake in the preheated oven at 350F for 25 minutes.
4. Serve the gratin right away.

Nutrition Info: Per Serving:Calories:414 Fat:25.9g
Protein:41.0g Carbohydrates:6.1g

Chicken Souvlaki

Servings: 4-6

Cooking Time: 12-15 Minutes

Ingredients:
- 4-6 chicken breasts, boneless, skinless
- For the marinade:
- 1 tablespoon dried oregano (use Greek or Turkish oregano)
- 1 tablespoon garlic, finely minced (or garlic puree from a jar) 1 tablespoon red wine vinegar
- 1 teaspoon dried thyme
- 1/2 cup lemon juice, freshly squeezed
- 1/2 cup olive oil

Directions:

1. If there are any visible fat on the chicken, trim them off. Cut each breasts into 5-6 pieces 1-inch thick crosswise strips. Put them in a Ziploc bag or a container with tight lid.

2. Whisk the marinade ingredients together until combined. Pour into the bag or container with the chicken, seal, and shake the bag or the container to coat the chicken. Marinade for 6 to 8 hours or more in the refrigerator.

3. When marinated, remove the chicken from the fridge, let thaw to room temperature, and drain; discard the marinade. Thread the chicken strips into skewers, about 6

pieces on each skewer, the meat folded over to it would not spin around on the skewers.

4. Mist the grill with olive oil. Preheat the charcoal or gas grill to medium high.

5. Grill the skewers for about 12-15 minutes, turning once as soon as you see grill marks. Souvlaki is done when the chicken is slightly browned and firm, but not hard to the touch.

Nutrition Info:Per Serving:360 cal., 26 g total fat (4.5 g sat fat), 90 mg chol., 170 mg sodium, 570 mg potassium, 3 g carb., 0 g fiber, <1 g sugar, and 30 g protein.

Rosemary Roasted New Potatoes

Servings: 6

Cooking Time: 1 Hour

Ingredients:

- 2 pounds new potatoes, washed
- 3 tablespoons olive oil
- 2 rosemary sprigs
- 4 garlic cloves, crushed
- Salt and pepper to taste

Directions:

1. Place the new potatoes in a large pot and cover them with water. Cook for 15 minutes then drain well.
2. Heat the oil in a skillet and add the rosemary and garlic.
3. Stir in the potatoes and continue cooking on medium flame for 20 minutes or until evenly golden brown.
4. Serve the potatoes warm.

Nutrition Info: Per Serving:Calories:168 Fat:7.2g Protein:2.7g Carbohydrates:24.6g

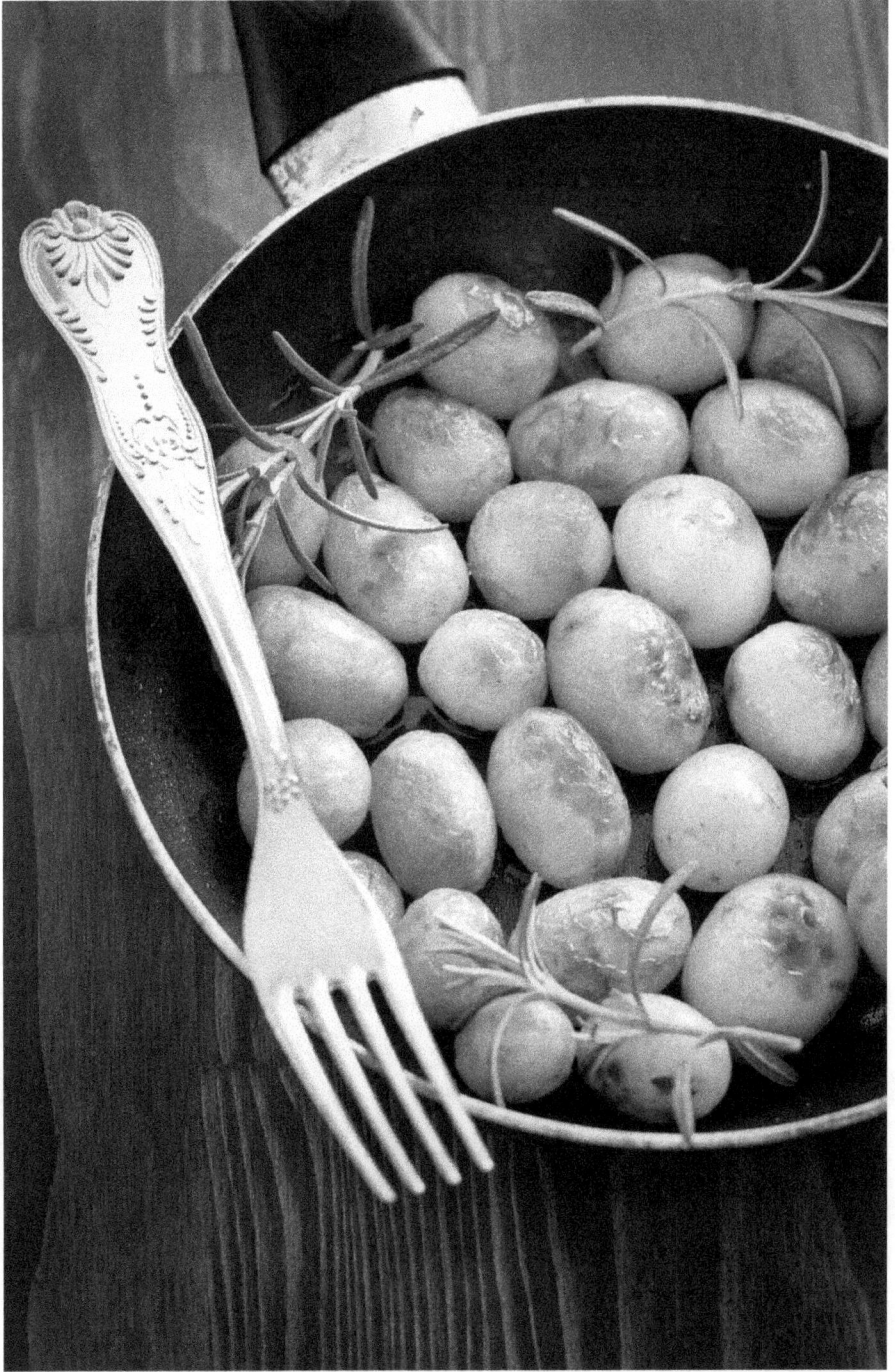

Artichoke Feta Penne

Servings: 4
Cooking Time: 40 Minutes

Ingredients:
- 8 oz. penne pasta
- 2 tablespoons olive oil
- 1 shallot, chopped
- 4 garlic cloves, chopped
- 1 jar artichoke hearts, drained and chopped
- 1 cup diced tomatoes
- ¼ cup white wine
- ½ cup vegetable stock
- Salt and pepper to taste
- 4 oz. feta cheese, crumbled

Directions:
1. Heat the oil in a skillet and stir in the shallot and garlic. Cook for 2
minutes until softened.
2. Add the artichoke hearts, tomatoes, wine and stock, as well as salt and pepper to taste.
3. Cook on low heat for 15 minutes.
4. In the meantime, cook the penne in a large pot of water until al dente, not more than 8 minutes.
5. Drain the pasta well and mix it with the artichoke sauce.

6. Serve the penne with crumbled feta cheese.

Nutrition Info: Per Serving:Calories:325 Fat:14.4g
Protein:11.1g Carbohydrates:35.8g

Grilled Chicken And Rustic Mustard Cream

Servings: 4
Cooking Time: 12 Minutes

Ingredients:
- 1 tablespoon plus 1 teaspoon whole-grain Dijon mustard, divided 1 tablespoon water
- 1 teaspoon fresh rosemary, chopped
- 1/4 teaspoon black pepper
- 1/4 teaspoon of salt
- 1 tablespoon olive oil
- 3 tablespoons light mayonnaise
- 4 pieces (6-ounces each) chicken breast halves, skinless, boneless Rosemary sprigs (optional)
- Cooking spray

Directions:
1. Preheat the grill.
2. In a small-sized bowl, combine the olive oil, 1-teaspoon of mustard; brush evenly over each chicken breast.
3. Coat the grill rack with the cooking spray, place and chicken, and grill for 6 minutes per side or until cooked.
4. While the chicken is grilling, combine the mayonnaise, the 1 tablespoon of mustard, and the water in a bowl.

5. Serve the grilled chicken with the mustard cream. If desired garnish with some rosemary sprigs.

Nutrition Info:Per Serving:262 Cal, 10 g total fat (1 g sat. fat, 4 g mono fat, 3 g poly fat), 39.6 g protein, 1.7 g carb.,0.2 g fiber, 102 mg chol., 1.4 mg iron, 448 mg sodium, and 25 mg calcium.

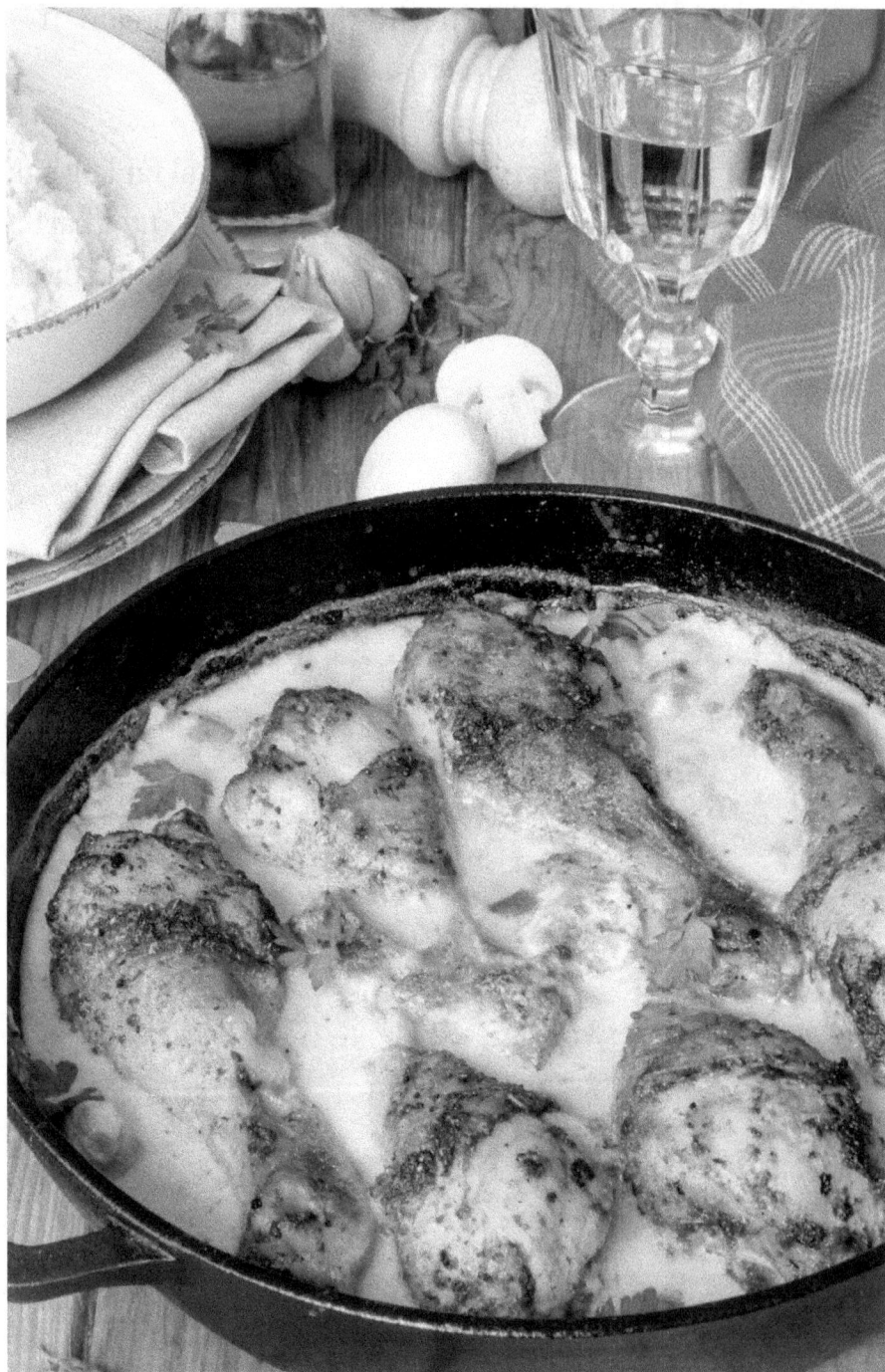

Balsamic Steak With Feta, Tomato, And Basil

Servings: 4
Cooking Time: 23 Minutes

Ingredients:

- 1 tablespoon balsamic vinegar
- 1/4 cup basil leaves
- 175 g Greek fetta, crumbled
- 2 tablespoons olive oil
- 2 teaspoons baby capers
- 4 sirloin steaks, trimmed
- 4 whole garlic cloves, skin on
- 6 roma tomatoes, halved
- Olive oil spray
- Salt and cracked black pepper

Directions:

1. Preheat the oven to 200C.
2. Line a baking tray with baking paper. Place the tomatoes and then scatter with the capers, crumbled feta, and the garlic cloves. Drizzle with 1 tablespoon of the olive oil and season with salt and pepper; cook for about 15 minutes or until the tomatoes are soft. Remove from the oven, set aside.

3. In a large non-metallic bowl, toss the steak with the remaining 1 tablespoon of olive oil, vinegar, salt and pepper; cover and refrigerate for 5 minutes.

4. Preheat the grill pan to high heat; grill the steaks for about 4 minutes per side or until cooked to your preference.

5. Serve with the prepared tomato mixture and sprinkle with basil.

Nutrition Info:Per Serving:520.3 Cal, 30 g total fat (12 g sat. fat), 3 g carb., 2 g fiber, 2 g sugar, 59 g protein, and 622.82 mg sodium.

Fried Chicken With Tzatziki Sauce

Servings: 4
Cooking Time: 45 Minutes

Ingredients:

- 4 chicken breasts, cubed
- 4 tablespoons olive oil
- 1 teaspoon dried basil
- 1 teaspoon dried oregano
- ½ teaspoon chili flakes
- Salt and pepper to taste
- 1 cup Greek yogurt
- 1 cucumber, grated
- 4 garlic cloves, minced
- 1 teaspoon lemon juice
- 1 teaspoon chopped mint
- 2 tablespoons chopped parsley

Directions:

1. Season the chicken with salt, pepper, basil, oregano and chili.
2. Heat the oil in a skillet and add the chicken. Cook on each side for 5 minutes on high heat just until golden brown.
3. Cover the chicken with a lid and continue cooking for 15-20 more minutes.

4. For the sauce, mix the yogurt, cucumber, garlic, lemon juice, mint and parsley, as well as salt and pepper.

5. Serve the chicken and the sauce fresh.

Nutrition Info: Per Serving:Calories:366 Fat:22.6g Protein:34.8g Carbohydrates:6.2g

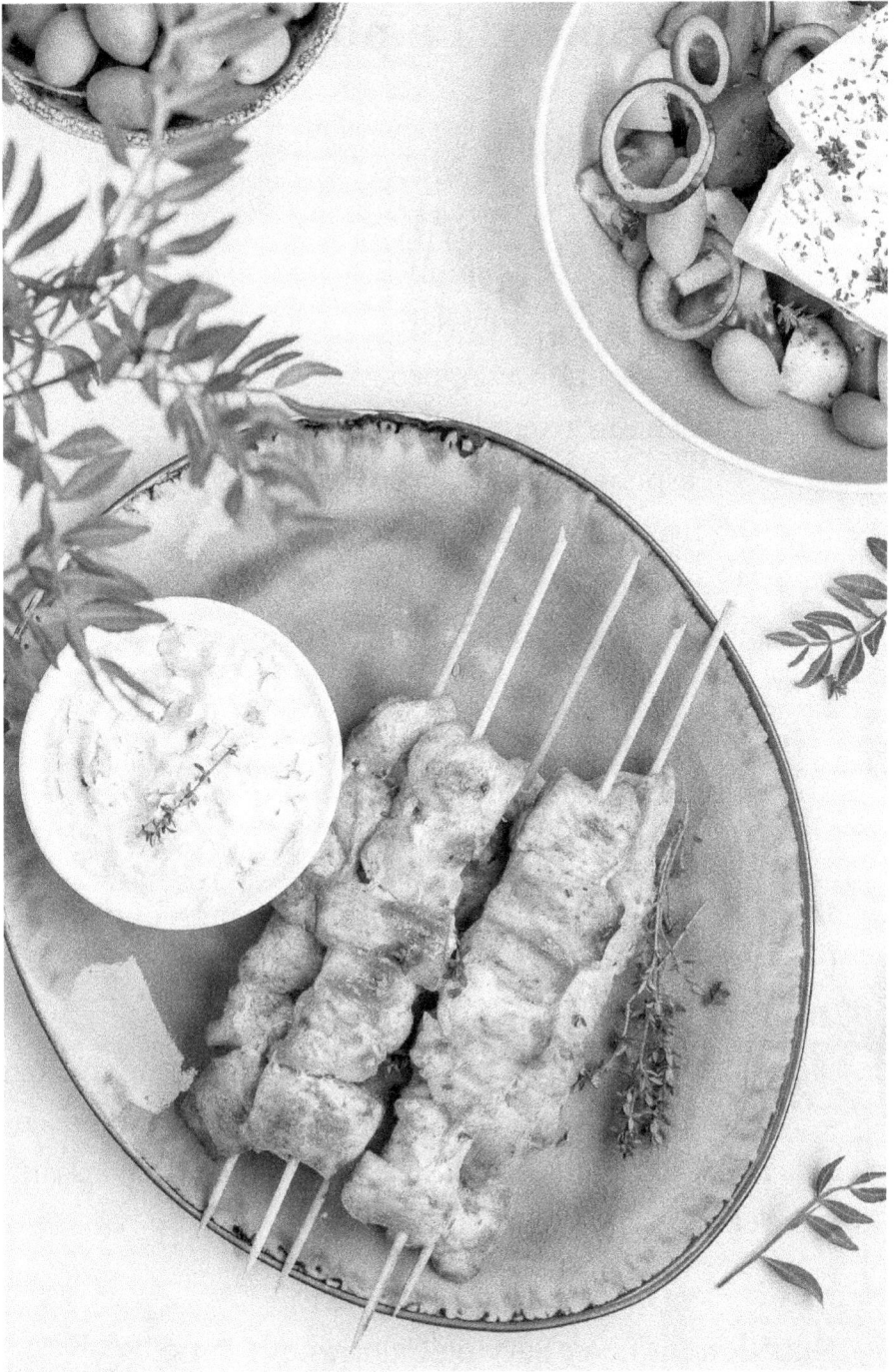

Spiced Lamb Patties

Servings: 8

Cooking Time: 1 Hour

Ingredients:

- 2 pounds ground lamb
- 4 garlic cloves, minced
- 1 shallot, finely chopped
- 1 teaspoon ground coriander
- 1 teaspoon ground cumin
- ½ teaspoon chili powder
- 1 teaspoon dried mint
- 2 tablespoons pine nuts, crushed
- Salt and pepper to taste
- 2 tablespoons chopped parsley
- 1 tablespoon chopped cilantro

Directions:

1. Mix the lamb meat and the remaining ingredients in a bowl.

2. Add salt and pepper and mix well.

3. Form small patties and place them on a chopping board.

4. Heat a grill pan over medium flame and cook on each side for 4-5 minutes or until browned and the juices run out clean.

5. Serve the patties warm.

Nutrition Info: Per Serving:Calories:231 Fat:9.9g Protein:32.4g Carbohydrates:1.3g

Chicken And Orzo Soup

Servings: 4
Cooking Time: 11 Minutes

Ingredients:
- ½ cup carrot, chopped
- 1 yellow onion, chopped
- 12 cups chicken stock
- 2 cups kale, chopped
- 3 cups chicken meat, cooked and shredded
- 1 cup orzo
- ¼ cup lemon juice
- 1 tablespoon olive oil

Directions:
1. Heat up a pot with the oil over medium heat, add the onion and sauté for 3 minutes.
2. Add the carrots and the rest of the ingredients, stir, bring to a simmer and cook for 8 minutes more.
3. Ladle into bowls and serve hot.

Nutrition Info: calories 300, fat 12.2, fiber 5.4, carbs 16.5, protein 12.2

Sweet And Sour Chicken Fillets

Servings: 4

Cooking Time: 40 Minutes

Ingredients:

- 4 chicken fillets
- 3 tablespoons olive oil
- 1 red pepper, sliced
- 1 lemon, juiced
- 1 tablespoon honey
- Salt and pepper to taste
- Chopped parsley for serving

Directions:

1. Season the chicken with salt and pepper.
2. Heat the oil in a skillet and add the chicken.
3. Cook on each side for 10 minutes.
4. Add the red pepper, lemon juice and honey and cook just for 1 additional minute.
5. Serve the chicken and the sauce warm and fresh.

Nutrition Info: Per Serving:Calories:309 Fat:18.0g Protein:29.4g Carbohydrates:7.5g

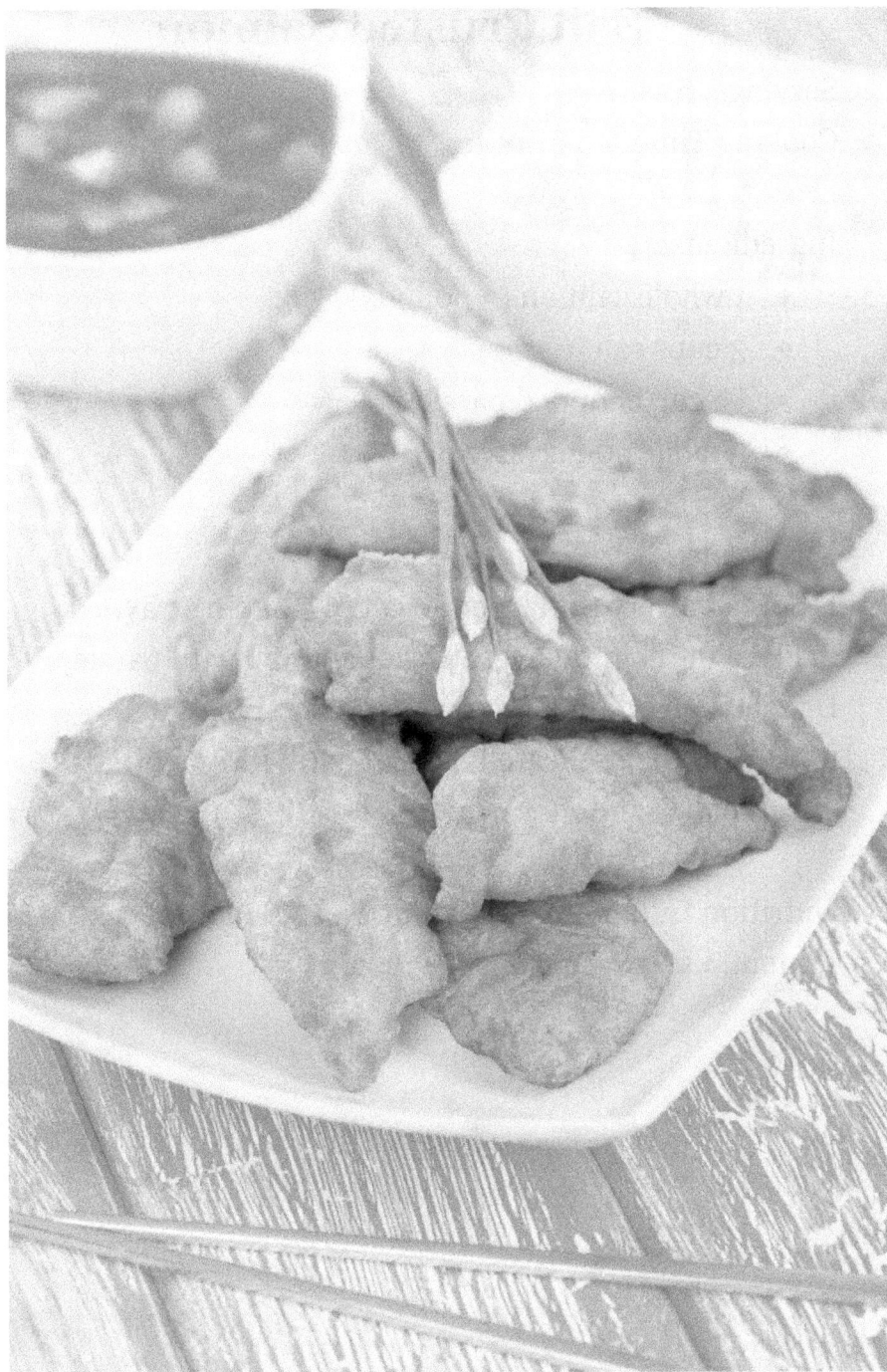

Salt Crusted Salmon

Servings: 6

Cooking Time: 40 Minutes

Ingredients:

- 1 whole salmon (3 pounds)
- 3 cups salt
- ½ cup chopped parsley
- 3 tablespoons olive oil

Directions:

1. Spread a very thin layer of salt in a baking tray.

2. Place the salmon over the salt and top with parsley. Drizzle with oil then top with the rest of the salt.

3. Cook in the preheated oven at 350F for 30 minutes.

4. Serve the salmon warm.

Nutrition Info: Per Serving:Calories:362 Fat:21.0g Protein:44.1g Carbohydrates:0.3g

Sun-dried Tomato Pesto Penne

Servings: 4

Cooking Time: 20 Minutes

Ingredients:

- 8 oz. penne
- ½ cup sun-dried tomatoes, drained well
- 2 tablespoons olive oil
- 4 garlic cloves, minced
- 2 tablespoons lemon juice
- 2 tablespoons pine nuts
- 2 tablespoons grated Parmesan cheese
- 1 pinch chili flakes

Directions:

1. Cook the penne in a large pot of salty water for 8 minutes or as long as it says on the package, just until al dente.
2. Drain the penne well.
3. For the pesto, combine the remaining ingredients in a blender and pulse until well mixed and smooth.
4. Mix the pesto with the penne and serve right away.

Nutrition Info: Per Serving:Calories:308 Fat:14.4g Protein:11.9g Carbohydrates:34.1g

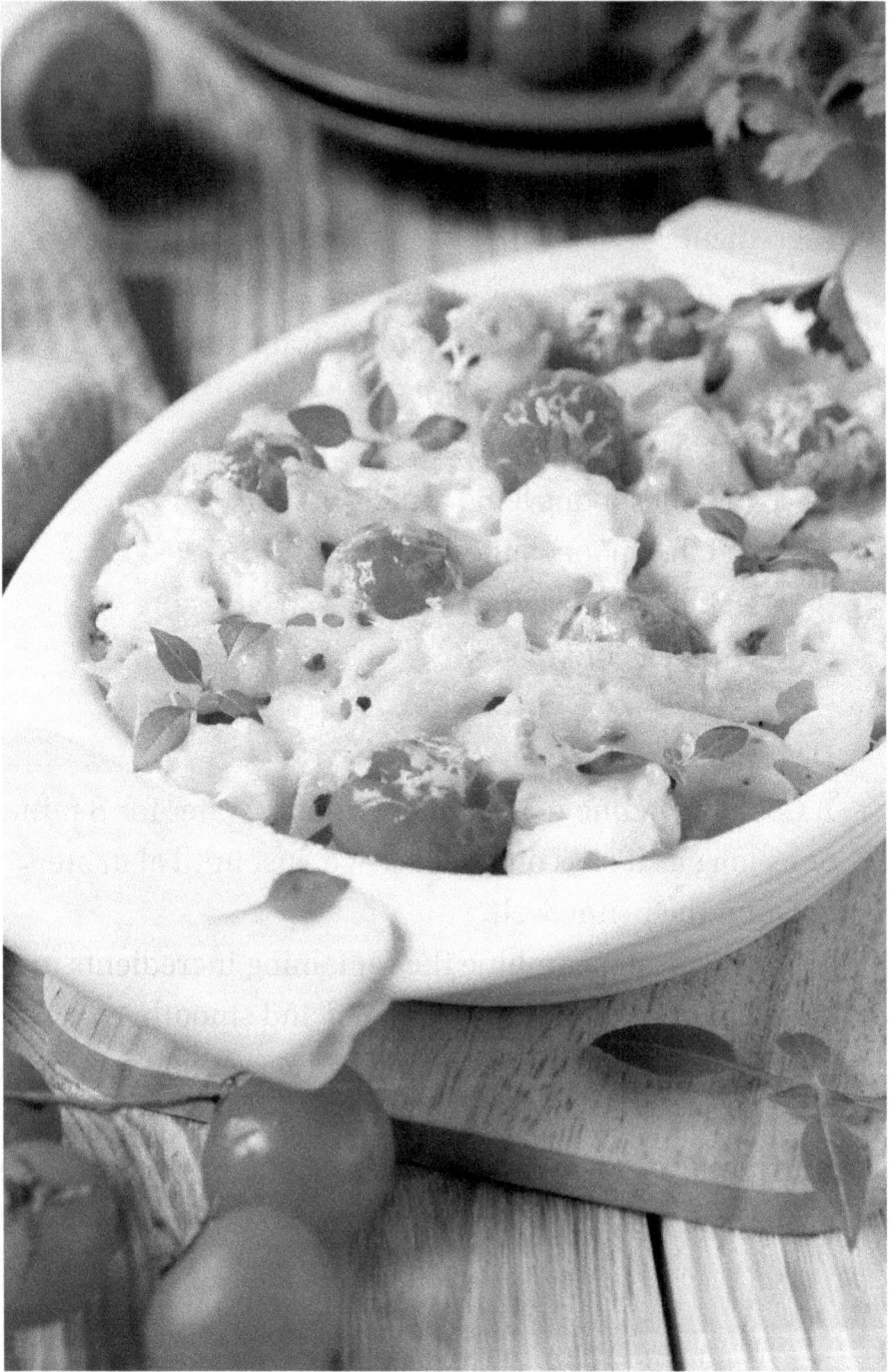

Herbed Marinated Sardines

Servings: 4

Cooking Time: 50 Minutes

Ingredients:
- 8 sardines
- ½ cup chopped parsley
- 2 tablespoons chopped cilantro
- 2 tablespoons pesto sauce
- 2 tablespoons olive oil
- 2 garlic cloves
- Salt and pepper to taste
- 2 tablespoons lemon juice

Directions:

1. Combine the herbs, pesto, oil, garlic, salt and pepper in a blender and pulse until smooth.

2. Spread the herb mixture over the sardines and season with salt and pepper.

3. Place the sardines in the fridge for 30 minutes.

4. Heat a grill pan over medium flame and place the sardines on the grill.

5. Cook on each side for 5-7 minutes.

6. Serve the sardines warm and fresh with your favorite side dish.

Nutrition Info: Per Serving:Calories:201 Fat:15.9g Protein:13.0g Carbohydrates:1.7g

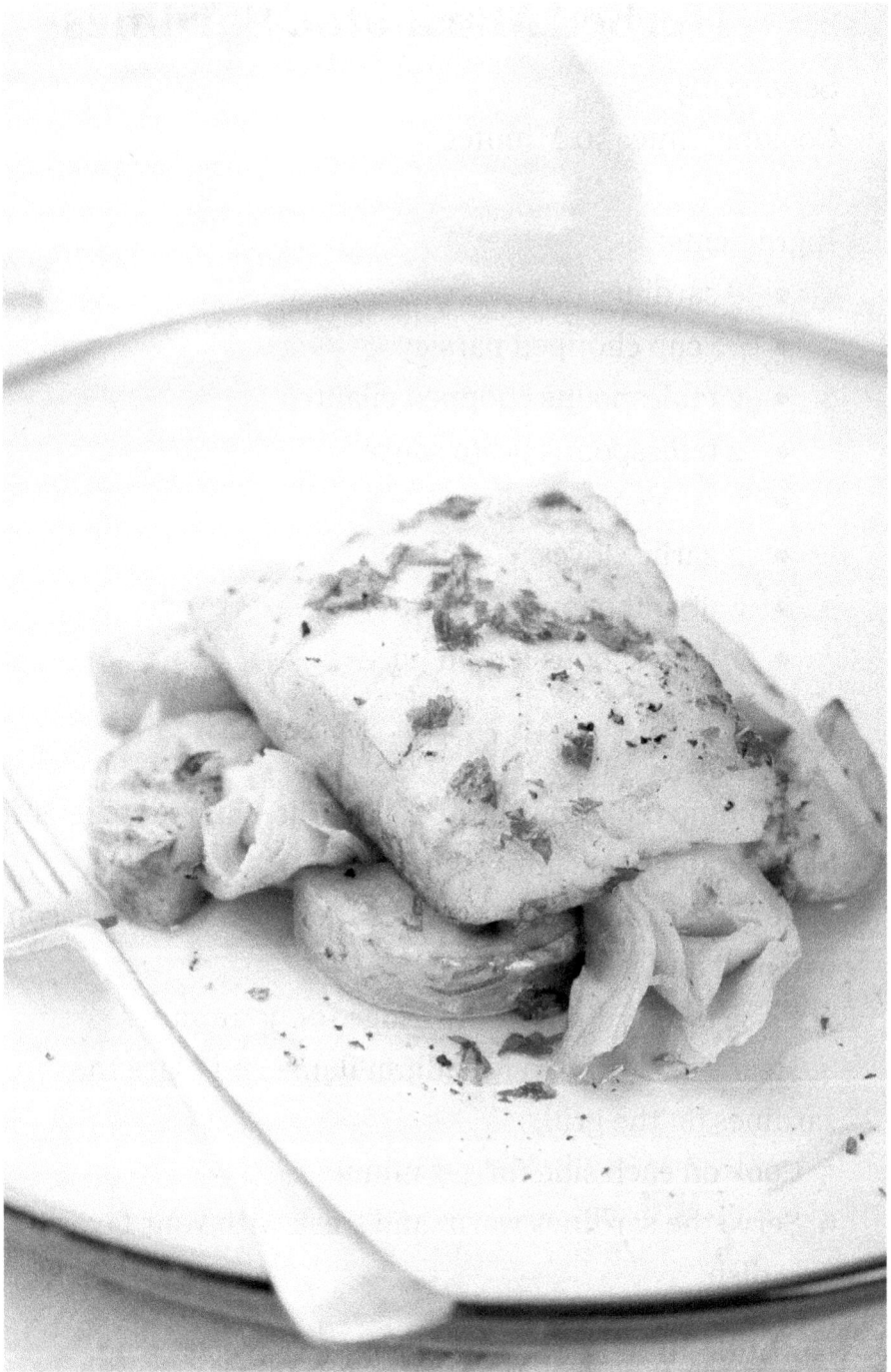

Spicy Tomato Poached Eggs

Servings: 4

Cooking Time: 30 Minutes

Ingredients:

- 2 tablespoons olive oil
- 2 shallots, chopped
- 2 garlic cloves, chopped
- 2 red bell peppers, cored and sliced
- 2 yellow bell peppers, cored and sliced
- 2 tomatoes, peeled and diced
- 1 cup vegetable stock
- 1 jalapeno, chopped
- Salt and pepper to taste
- 4 eggs

Directions:

1. Heat the oil in a saucepan and stir in the shallots, garlic, bell peppers and jalapeno. Cook for 5 minutes.
2. Add the tomatoes, stock, thyme and bay leaf, as well as salt and pepper to taste.
3. Cook for 10 minutes on low heat.
4. Crack open the eggs and drop them in the hot sauce.
5. Cook on low heat for 5 additional minutes.
6. Serve the eggs and the sauce fresh and warm.

Nutrition Info: Per Serving:Calories:179 Fat:11.9g
Protein:7.6g Carbohydrates:11.7g

Mediterranean Scones

Servings: 8
Cooking Time: 15-20 Minutes

Ingredients:
- 1 egg, beaten, to glaze
- 1 tablespoon baking powder
- 1 tablespoon olive oil
- 1/4 tsp salt
- 10 black olives, pitted, halved
- 100 g feta cheese, cubed
- 300 ml full-fat milk
- 350 g self-rising whole-wheat flour
- 50 g butter, cut in pieces
- 8 halves Italian sundried tomatoes, coarsely chopped

Directions:
1. Preheat the oven to 220C, gas to 7, or fan to 200C.
2. Grease a large-sized baking sheet with butter.
3. In a large mixing bowl, mix the flour, the baking powder, and the salt. Rub in the oil and the butter, until the flour mix resembles fine crumbs. Add the cheese, tomatoes, and the olives.
4. Create a well in the center of the flour mix, pour the milk, and with a knife, mix using cutting movements, until the flour mixture is a stickyish, soft dough. Make sure that you do not over mix the dough.

5. Flour the work surface and your hands well; shape the dough into 3 to 4- cm think round. Cut into 8 wedges; place the wedges well apart in the
prepared baking sheet. Brush the wedges with the beaten egg; bake for about 15-20 minutes, until the dough has risen, golden, and springy.
6. Transfer into a wire rack; cover with a clean tea towel to keep them soft.
7. Serve warm and buttered.
8. Store in airtight container for up to 2 to 3 days.

Nutrition Info:Per Serving:293 Cal, 14 g total fat (7 g sat. fat), 36 g carb.,0 g sugar, 2 g fiber, 8 g protein, and 2 g sodium.

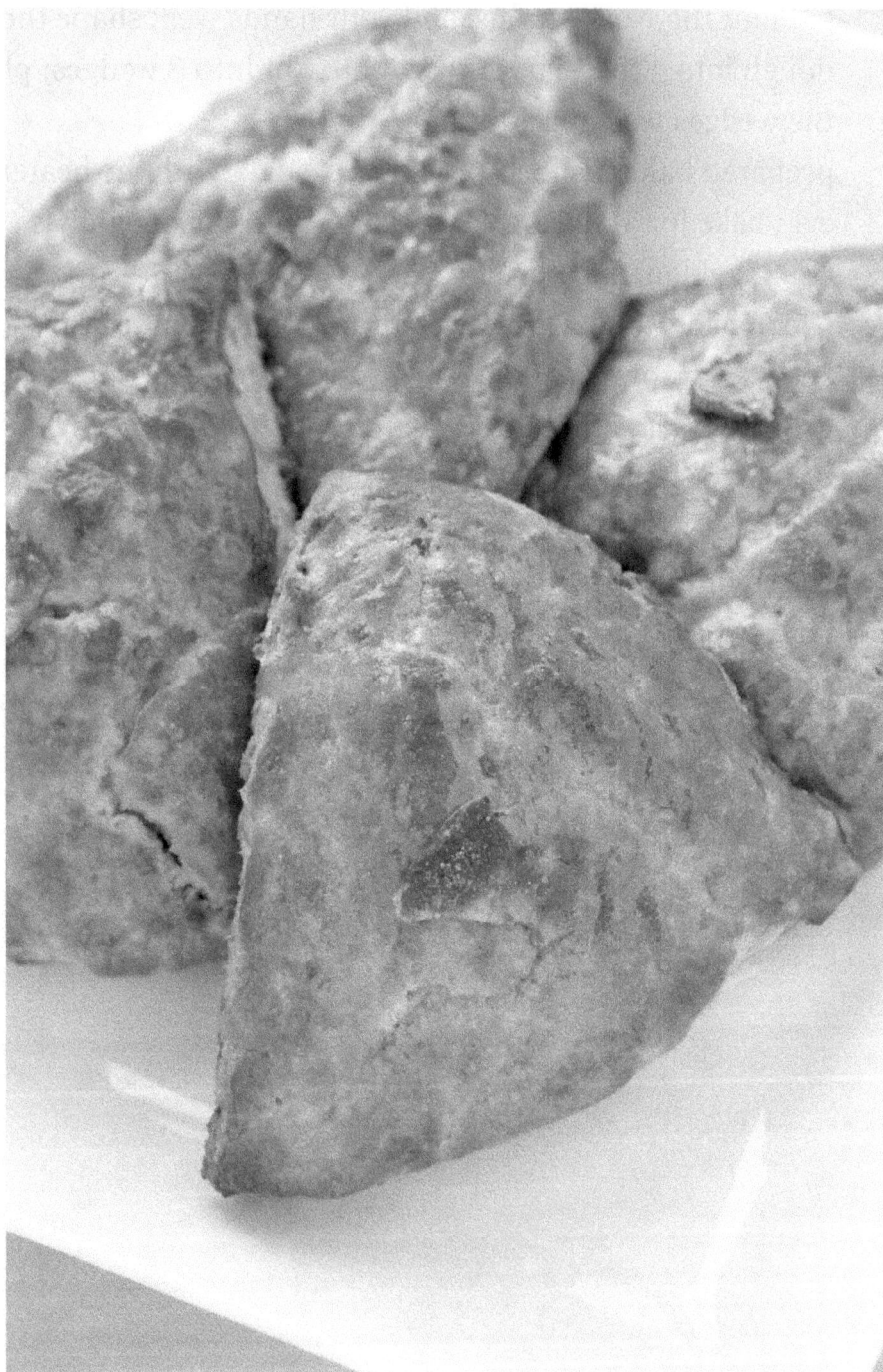

Mixed Olives Braised Chicken

Servings: 4

Cooking Time: 1 Hour

Ingredients:

- 4 chicken breasts
- 2 shallots, sliced
- 4 garlic cloves, chopped
- 2 red bell peppers, cored and sliced
- ½ cup black olives
- ½ cup green olives
- ½ cup kalamata olives
- 2 tablespoons olive oil
- ¼ cup white wine
- ½ cup vegetable stock
- Salt and pepper to taste
- 1 bay leaf
- 1 thyme sprig

Directions:

1. Combine the shallots, garlic, bell peppers, olives, oil, wine and stock in a deep dish baking pan.
2. Season with salt and pepper and place the chicken in the pan over the olives.
3. Cook in the preheated oven at 350F for 45 minutes.
4. Serve the chicken warm and fresh.

Nutrition Info: Per Serving:Calories:280 Fat:16.3g Protein:22.9g Carbohydrates:7.9g

Coconut Chicken Meatballs

Servings: 4

Cooking Time: 10 Minutes

Ingredients:

- 2 cups ground chicken
- 1 teaspoon minced garlic
- 1 teaspoon dried dill
- 1/3 carrot, grated
- 1 egg, beaten
- 1 tablespoon olive oil
- ¼ cup coconut flakes
- ½ teaspoon salt

Directions:

1. In the mixing bowl mix up together ground chicken, minced garlic, dried dill, carrot, egg, and salt.
2. Stir the chicken mixture with the help of the fingertips until homogenous.
3. Then make medium balls from the mixture.
4. Coat every chicken ball in coconut flakes.
5. Heat up olive oil in the skillet.
6. Add chicken balls and cook them for 3 minutes from each side. The cooked chicken balls will have a golden brown color.

Nutrition Info:Per Serving:calories 200, fat 11.5, fiber 0.6, carbs 1.7, protein 21.9

Grilled Turkey With White Bean Mash

Servings: 4

Cooking Time: 45 Minutes

Ingredients:

- 4 turkey breast fillets
- 1 teaspoon chili powder
- 1 teaspoon dried parsley
- Salt and pepper to taste
- 2 cans white beans, drained
- 4 garlic cloves, minced
- 2 tablespoons lemon juice
- 3 tablespoons olive oil
- 2 sweet onions, sliced
- 2 tablespoons tomato paste

Directions:

1. Season the turkey with salt, pepper and dried parsley.
2. Heat a grill pan over medium flame and place the turkey on the grill. Cook on each side for 7 minutes.
3. For the mash, combine the beans, garlic, lemon juice, salt and pepper in a blender and pulse until well mixed and smooth.
4. Heat the oil in a skillet and add the onions. Cook for 10 minutes until caramelized. Add the tomato paste and cook

for 2 more minutes. 5. Serve the grilled turkey with bean mash and caramelized onions.

Nutrition Info: Per Serving:Calories:337 Fat:8.2g Protein:21.1g Carbohydrates:47.2g

Vegetable Turkey Casserole

Servings: 8

Cooking Time: 1 ¼ Hours

Ingredients:

- 3 tablespoons olive oil
- 2 pounds turkey breasts, cubed
- 1 sweet onion, chopped
- 3 carrots, sliced
- 2 celery stalks, sliced
- 2 garlic cloves, chopped
- ½ teaspoon cumin powder
- ½ teaspoon dried thyme
- 2 cans diced tomatoes
- 1 cup chicken stock
- 1 bay leaf
- Salt and pepper to taste

Directions:

1. Heat the oil in a deep heavy pot and stir in the turkey.

2. Cook for 5 minutes until golden on all sides then add the onion, carrot, celery and garlic. Cook for 5 more minutes then add the rest of the ingredients.

3. Season with salt and pepper and cook in the preheated oven at 350F for 40 minutes.

4. Serve the casserole warm and fresh.

Nutrition Info: Per Serving:Calories:186 Fat:7.3g Protein:20.1g Carbohydrates:9.9g

Mediterranean Grilled Pork With Tomato Salsa

Servings: 4

Cooking Time: 1 Hour

Ingredients:

- 4 pork chops
- 1 teaspoon dried oregano
- 1 teaspoon dried basil
- 1 teaspoon dried marjoram
- Salt and pepper to taste
- 4 tomatoes, peeled and diced
- 1 jalapeno, chopped
- 1 shallot, chopped
- 2 garlic cloves, minced
- 1 green onion, chopped
- 2 tablespoons chopped parsley
- 1 tablespoon lemon juice

Directions:

1. Season with salt and pepper, oregano, basil and marjoram.
2. Heat a grill pan over medium flame and place the pork chops on the grill.
3. Cook on each side for 5-6 minutes.

4. For the salsa, mix the tomatoes, jalapeno, shallot, garlic, onion and parsley. Add salt and pepper to taste. Add the lemon juice as well.

5. Serve the pork chops with salsa.

Nutrition Info: Per Serving:Calories:286 Fat:20.3g Protein:19.4g Carbohydrates:6.3g

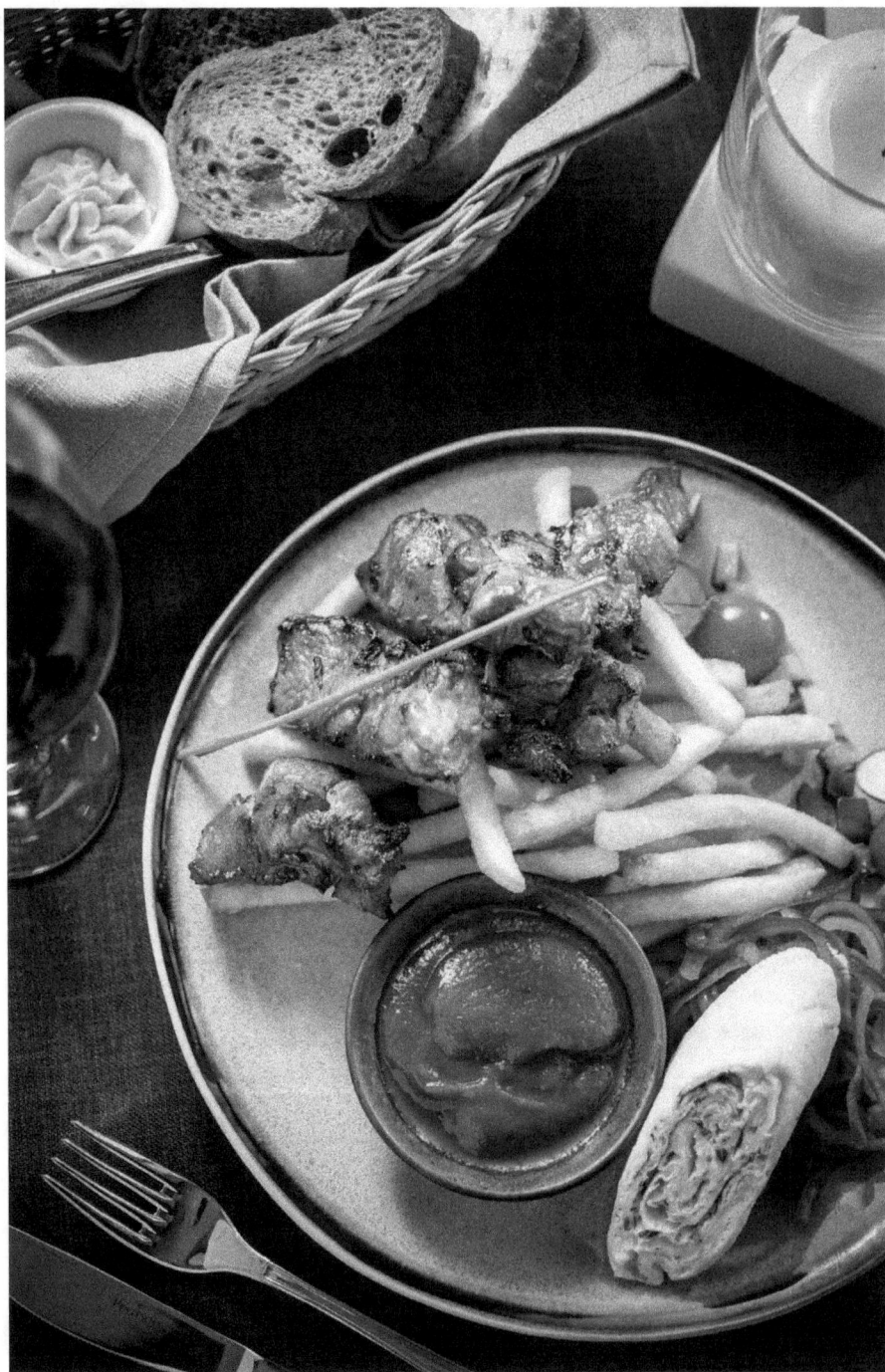

Beef And Macaroni Soup

Servings: 6

Cooking Time: 30 Minutes

Ingredients:

- ½ cup elbow macaroni
- 1 teaspoon coconut oil
- 1/3 teaspoon minced garlic
- 2 oz yellow onion, diced
- 1 ½ cup ground beef
- ½ teaspoon dried oregano
- ½ teaspoon dried thyme
- 1 teaspoon salt
- 1 teaspoon chili flakes
- 3 oz Mozzarella, shredded
- 1 teaspoon dried basil
- 5 cups beef broth
- 1 tablespoon cream cheese
- 1 cup water, for cooking macaroni

Directions:

1. Pour water in the pan and bring it to boil.
2. Add elbow macaroni and cook them according to the manufacturer directions.
3. Then drain water from the cooked elbow macaroni.
4. Put coconut oil in the big pot and melt it.

5. Add minced garlic, yellow onion, ground beef, dried oregano, dried thyme, salt, chili flakes, and dried basil.
6. Cook the ingredients for 10 minutes over the medium-low heat. Stir the mixture from time to time.
7. Add beef broth and cream cheese. Stir the soup until it is homogenous.
8. Cook the soup for 10 minutes.
9. Then add cooked elbow macaroni and stir well.
10. Bring the soup to boil and remove from the heat.
11. Ladle the cooked soup in the serving bowls and garnish with Mozzarella.

Nutrition Info:Per Serving:calories 180, fat 9.2, fiber 0.5, carbs 7.6, protein 15.7

Provencal Beef Stew

Servings: 8

Cooking Time: 1 ½ Hours

Ingredients:

- 3 tablespoons olive oil
- 2 pounds beef roast, cubed
- 2 sweet onions, chopped
- 4 garlic cloves, chopped
- 2 carrots, diced
- 2 celery stalks, diced
- 1 can diced tomatoes
- 2 tomatoes, peeled and diced
- 1 cup vegetable stock
- 1 jalapeno, chopped
- 1 bay leaf
- 1 thyme sprig
- Salt and pepper to taste

Directions:

1. Heat the oil in a skillet and stir in the beef. Cook for 10 minutes on all sides.

2. Add the onions and garlic and cook for 5 more minutes.

3. Stir in the remaining ingredients and season with salt and pepper.

4. Place a lid on and cook on low heat for 1 hour.

5. Serve the stew warm and fresh.

Nutrition Info: Per Serving:Calories:284 Fat:12.5g Protein:35.4g Carbohydrates:6.5g

Greek Beef Meatballs

Servings: 8

Cooking Time: 1 Hour

Ingredients:

- 2 pounds ground beef
- 6 garlic cloves, minced
- 1 teaspoon dried mint
- 1 teaspoon dried oregano
- 1 shallot, finely chopped
- 1 carrot, grated
- 1 egg
- 1 tablespoon tomato paste
- 3 tablespoons chopped parsley
- Salt and pepper to taste

Directions:

1. Combine all the ingredients in a bowl and mix well.
2. Season with salt and pepper then form small meatballs and place them in a baking tray lined with baking paper.
3. Bake in the preheated oven at 350F for 25 minutes.
4. Serve the meatballs warm and fresh.

Nutrition Info: Per Serving:Calories:229 Fat:7.7g Protein:35.5g Carbohydrates:2.4g

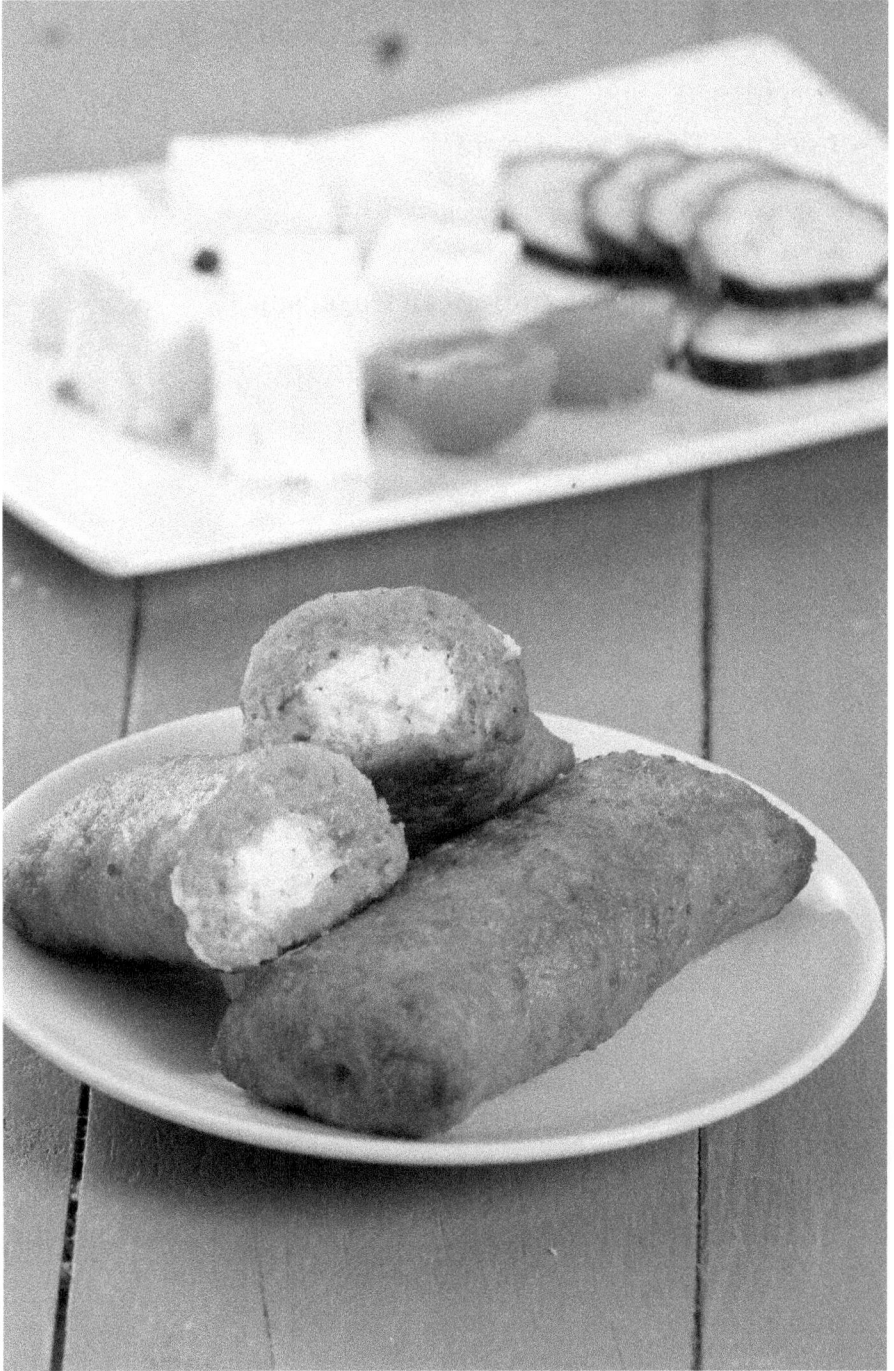

Sausage And Beans Soup

Servings: 4

Cooking Time: 20 Minutes

Ingredients:

- 1 pound Italian pork sausage, sliced
- ¼ cup olive oil
- 1 carrot, chopped
- 1 yellow onion, chopped
- 1 celery stalk, chopped
- 2 garlic cloves, minced
- ½ pound kale, chopped
- 4 cups chicken stock
- 28 ounces canned cannellini beans, drained and rinsed
- 1 bay leaf
- 1 teaspoon rosemary, dried
- Salt and black pepper to the taste
- ½ cup parmesan, grated

Directions:

1. Heat up a pot with the oil over medium heat, add the sausage and brown for 5 minutes.
2. Add the onion, carrots, garlic and celery and sauté for 3 minutes more.

3. Add the rest of the ingredients except the parmesan, bring to a simmer and cook over medium heat for 30 minutes.

4. Discard the bay leaf, ladle the soup into bowls, sprinkle the parmesan on top and serve.

Nutrition Info: calories 564, fat 26.5, fiber 15.4, carbs 37.4, protein 26.6

Jalapeno Grilled Salmon With Tomato Confit

Servings: 4

Cooking Time: 30 Minutes

Ingredients:
- 4 salmon fillets
- 1 jalapeno
- 4 garlic cloves
- 2 tablespoons tomato paste
- 2 tablespoons olive oil
- Salt and pepper to taste
- 2 cups cherry tomatoes, halved
- 1 shallot, chopped
- 1 tablespoon olive oil

Directions:

1. Combine the jalapeno, garlic, tomato paste and oil in a mortar. Mix well until a smooth paste is formed.

2. Spread the spicy paste over the salmon and season it with salt and pepper.

3. Heat a grill pan over medium flame then place the fish on the grill.

4. Cook on each side for 5-6 minutes.

5. For the confit, heat 1 tablespoon of oil in a skillet. Add the shallot and cook for 1 minute then stir in the cherry

tomatoes, salt and pepper. Cook for 2 minutes on high heat.

6. Serve the grilled salmon with the tomatoes.

Nutrition Info: Per Serving:Calories:237 Fat:14.5g Protein:24.0g Carbohydrates:4.4g

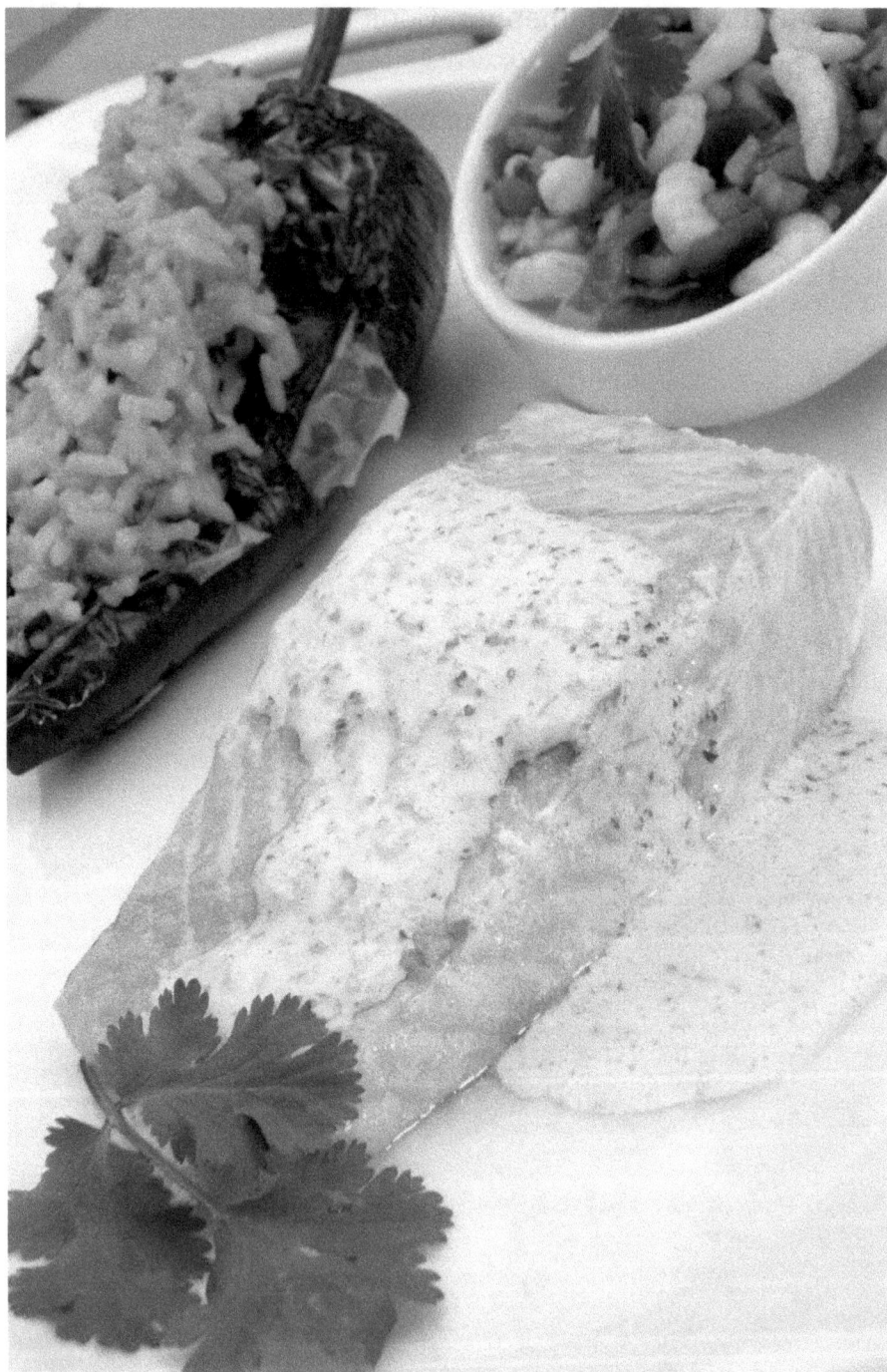

Chicken And Rice Soup

Servings: 4

Cooking Time: 35 Minutes

Ingredients:

- 6 cups chicken stock
- 1 and ½ cups chicken meat, cooked and shredded
- 1 bay leaf
- 1 yellow onion, chopped
- 2 tablespoons olive oil
- 1/3 cup white rice
- 1 egg, whisked
- Juice of ½ lemon
- 1 cup asparagus, trimmed and halved
- 1 cup carrots, chopped
- ½ cup dill, chopped
- Salt and black pepper to the taste

Directions:

1. Heat up a pot with the oil over medium heat, add the onions and sauté for 5 minutes.
2. Add the stock, dill, the rice and the bay leaf, stir, bring to a boil over medium heat and cook for 10 minutes.
3. Add the rest of the ingredients except the egg and the lemon juice, stir and cook for 15 minutes more.

4. Add the egg whisked with the lemon juice gradually, whisk the soup, cook for 2 minutes more, divide into bowls and serve.

Nutrition Info: calories 263, fat 18.5, fiber 4.5, carbs 19.8, protein 14.5

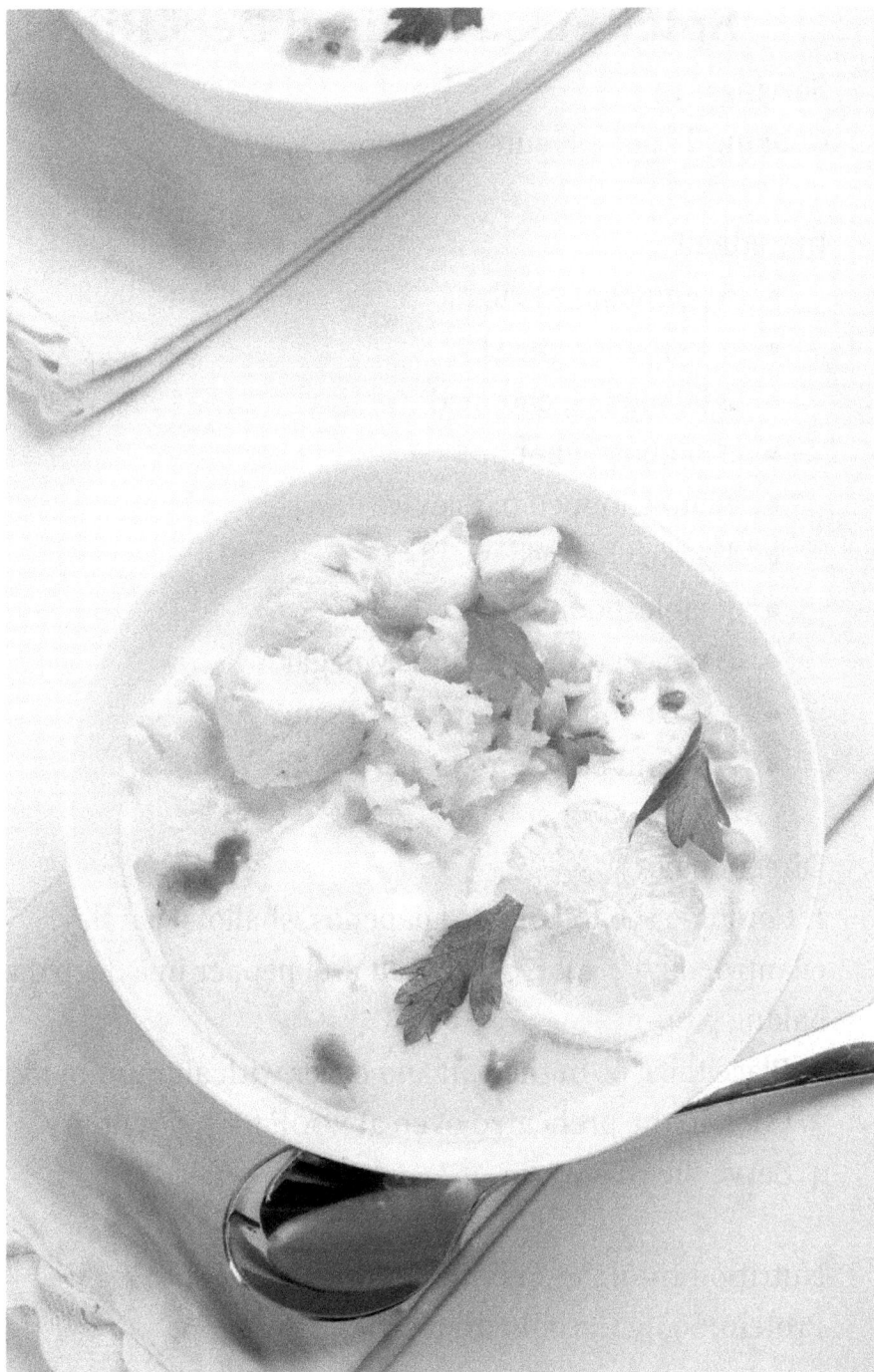

Spicy Salsa Braised Beef Ribs

Servings: 12
Cooking Time: 4 Hours

Ingredients:
- 6 pounds beef ribs
- 4 tomatoes, diced
- 2 jalapenos, chopped
- 2 shallots, chopped
- 1 cup chopped parsley
- ½ cup chopped cilantro
- 3 tablespoons olive oil
- 2 tablespoons balsamic vinegar
- 1 teaspoon Worcestershire sauce
- Salt and pepper to taste

Directions:
1. Combine the tomatoes, jalapenos, shallots, parsley, cilantro, oil, vinegar, sauce, salt and pepper in a deep dish baking pan.
2. Place the ribs in the pan and cover with aluminum foil.
3. Cook in the preheated oven at 300F for 3 1/3 hours.
4. Serve the ribs warm.

Nutrition Info: Per Serving:Calories:464 Fat:17.8g
Protein:69.4g Carbohydrates:2.5g

Pork And Prunes Stew

Servings: 8
Cooking Time: 1 ¼ Hours

Ingredients:

- 2 pounds pork tenderloin, cubed
- 2 tablespoons olive oil
- 1 sweet onions, chopped
- 4 garlic cloves, chopped
- 2 carrots, diced
- 2 celery stalks, chopped
- 2 tomatoes, peeled and diced
- 1 cup vegetable stock
- ½ cup white wine
- 1 pound prunes, pitted
- 1 bay leaf
- 1 thyme sprig
- 1 teaspoon mustard seeds
- 1 teaspoon coriander seeds
- Salt and pepper to taste

Directions:
1. Combine all the ingredients in a deep dish baking pan.
2. Add salt and pepper to taste and cook in the preheated oven at 350F for 1 hour, adding more liquid as it cooks if needed.

3. Serve the stew warm and fresh.

Nutrition Info: Per Serving:Calories:363 Fat:7.9g
Protein:31.7g Carbohydrates:41.4g

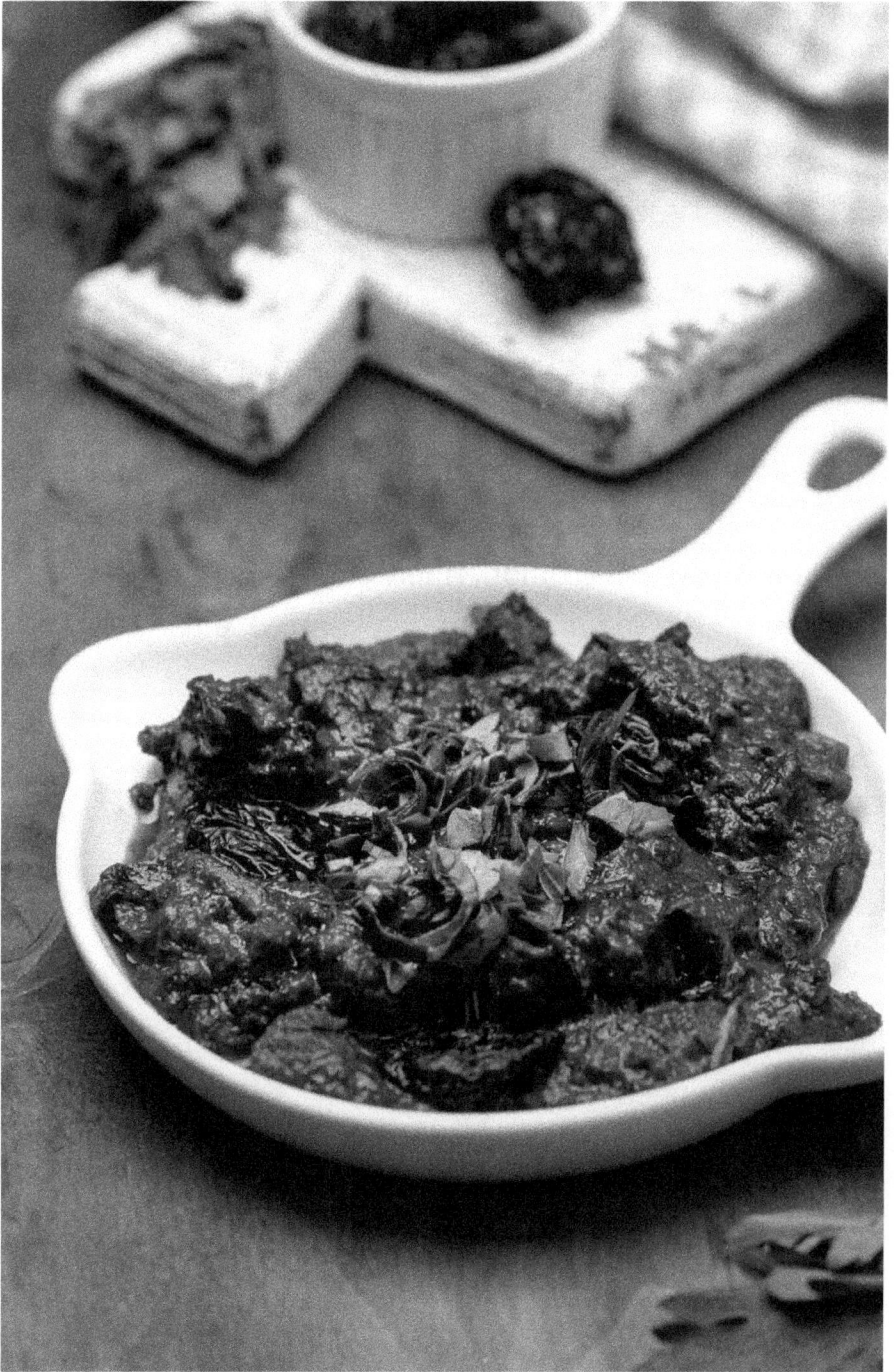

Low-carb And Paleo Mediterranean Zucchini Noodles

Servings: 4

Cooking Time: 10 Minutes

Ingredients:

- 4 medium (about 8 inches long) zucchini
- 3-4 garlic cloves, peeled
- 1 tablespoon olive oil (or slightly more if you have a lot of noodles) 2 tablespoons olive oil
- 1/4 cup red onion, finely chopped
- 1 tablespoon garlic, finely minced, plus
- 1/2 teaspoon dried oregano
- 1/2 teaspoon Italian herb blend
- Red pepper flakes, to taste (1/2 teaspoon, less or more)
- 1/4 cup parsley, chopped
- 2 cups cherry tomatoes, cut into halves
- 1/2 cup Kalamata olives, drained, cut in half (or regular black olives) 1/4 cup capers, drained, chopped

Directions:

1. Except for the zucchini, prepare and ready the rest of the ingredients.

2. Wash the zucchini well and pat dry with paper towel. Spiralize the noodles using a spiralizer. With a kitchen

shear, cut through the pile of zoodles (zucchini noodles) a few times to shorten them.

3. For the sauce:

4. In a medium-frying pan, heat the 2 tablespoons olive oil over medium high heat. Add the red onions; cook for 2 minutes. Add the minced garlic
and the dried herbs, cook for 1 minute. Add the tomatoes; cook for 2 minutes. Add the capers, olives, and red pepper flakes; cook for about 1-2 minutes. Turn the heat off; stir the parsley in to mix.

5. For the zoodles:

6. In a large-sized-sized nonstick wok or pan, heat the remaining 1 tablespoon olive oil. When hot, add the whole garlic cloves, cook for about 30 seconds, or just until fragrant, discard the garlic. Add the zoodles; cook for 2 to 3 minutes on high heat, stirring a couple of times, just until the zoodles are beginning to soften and hot.

7. Divide the zoodles between 4 bowls. Top each serve with a generous scoop of the sauce. Best when freshly made and served. However, if there are any leftovers, you can keep them in the fridge and reheat gently in a pan.

Nutrition Info:Per Serving:190 cal., 13 g total fat (1.5 g sat fat), 0 mg chol., 420 mg sodium, 8400 mg potassium, 16 g carb., 5 g fiber, 9 g sugar, and 4 g protein.

Pork And Rice Soup

Servings: 4

Cooking Time: 7 Hours

Ingredients:

- 2 pounds pork stew meat, cubed
- A pinch of salt and black pepper
- 6 cups water
- 1 leek, sliced
- 2 bay leaves
- 1 carrot, sliced
- 3 tablespoons olive oil
- 1 cup white rice
- 2 cups yellow onion, chopped
- ½ cup lemon juice
- 1 tablespoon cilantro, chopped

Directions:

1. In your slow cooker, combine the pork with the water and the rest of the ingredients except the cilantro, put the lid on and cook on Low for 7 hours.

2. Stir the soup, ladle into bowls, sprinkle the cilantro on top and serve.

Nutrition Info: calories 300, fat 15, fiber 7.6, carbs 17.4, protein 22.4

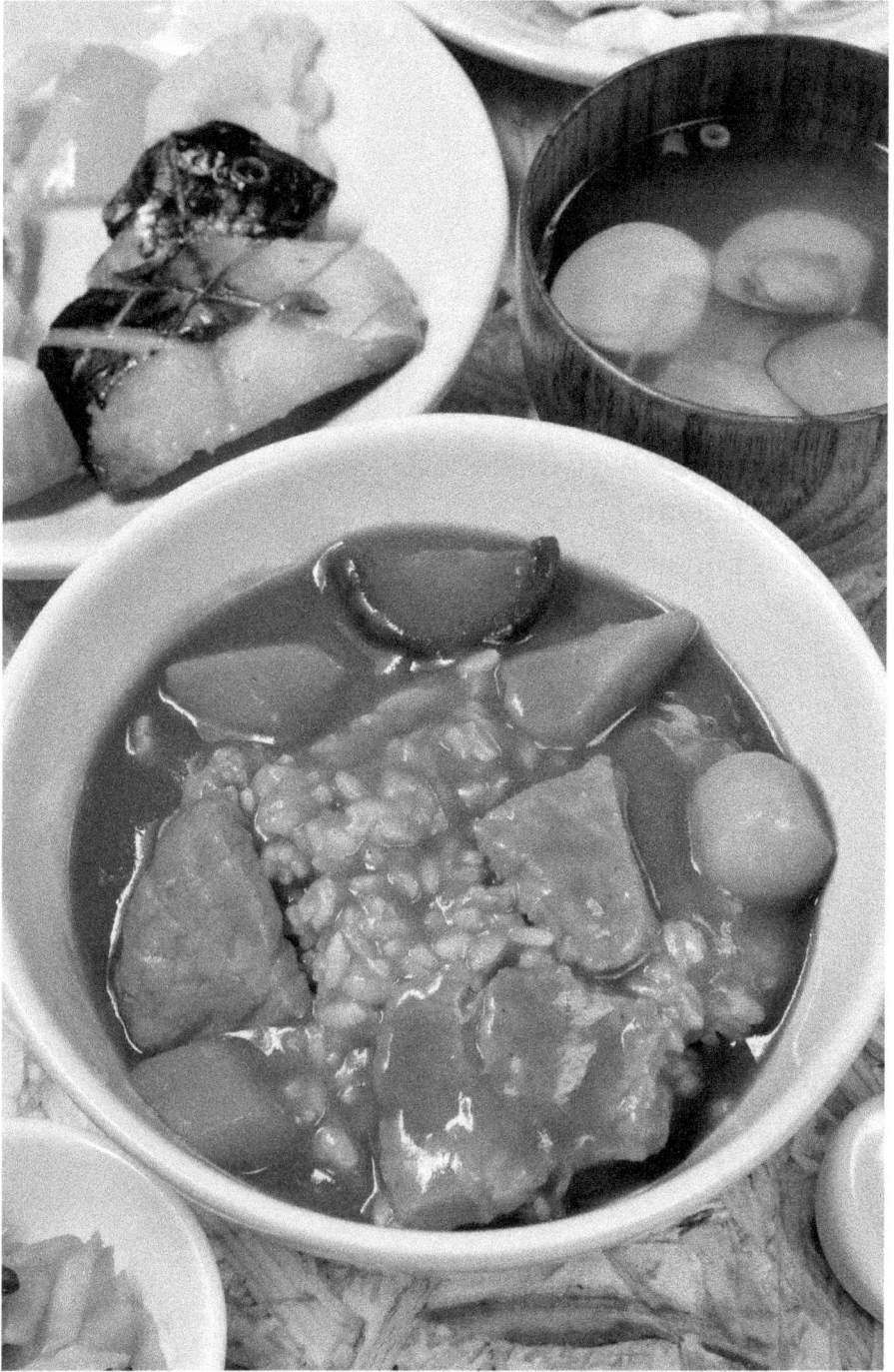

Tomato Roasted Feta

Servings: 4
Cooking Time: 45 Minutes

Ingredients:
- 8 oz. feta cheese
- 2 tomatoes, peeled and diced
- 2 garlic cloves, chopped
- 1 cup tomato juice
- 1 thyme sprig
- 1 oregano sprig

Directions:
1. Mix the tomatoes, garlic, tomato juice, thyme and oregano in a small deep dish baking pan.
2. Place the feta in the pan as well and cover with aluminum foil.
3. Cook in the preheated oven at 350F for 10 minutes.
4. Serve the feta and the sauce fresh.

Nutrition Info: Per Serving:Calories:173 Fat:12.2g Protein:9.2g Carbohydrates:7.8g

Fettuccine With Spinach And Shrimp

Servings: 4-6
Cooking Time: 10 Minutes

Ingredients:
- 8 ounces whole-wheat fettuccine pasta, uncooked
- 3 garlic cloves, peeled, chopped
- 2 teaspoons dried basil, crushed
- 12 ounces medium raw shrimp, peeled, deveined
- 1/4 teaspoon crushed red pepper flakes
- 1/2 cup crumbled feta cheese
- 1 teaspoon salt
- 1 package (10 ounce) frozen spinach, thawed
- 1 cup sour cream

Directions:
1. In a large-sized mixing bowl, combine sour cream, the feta, basil, garlic, salt, and red pepper.
2. According to the package instructions, cook the fettuccine. After the first 8 minutes of cooking, add the spinach and the shrimp to the boiling water with pasta; boil for 2 minutes more and then drain thoroughly.

3. Add the hot pasta, spinach, and shrimp mixture into the bowl with the sour cream mix; lightly toss and serve immediately.

Nutrition Info:Per Serving:417.9 Cal, 18 g total fat (9.8 g sat. fat), 197.6 mg chol., 1395.6 mg sodium, 39.7 g carb., 2.5 g fiber, 3.3 g sugar, and 25.2 g protein.

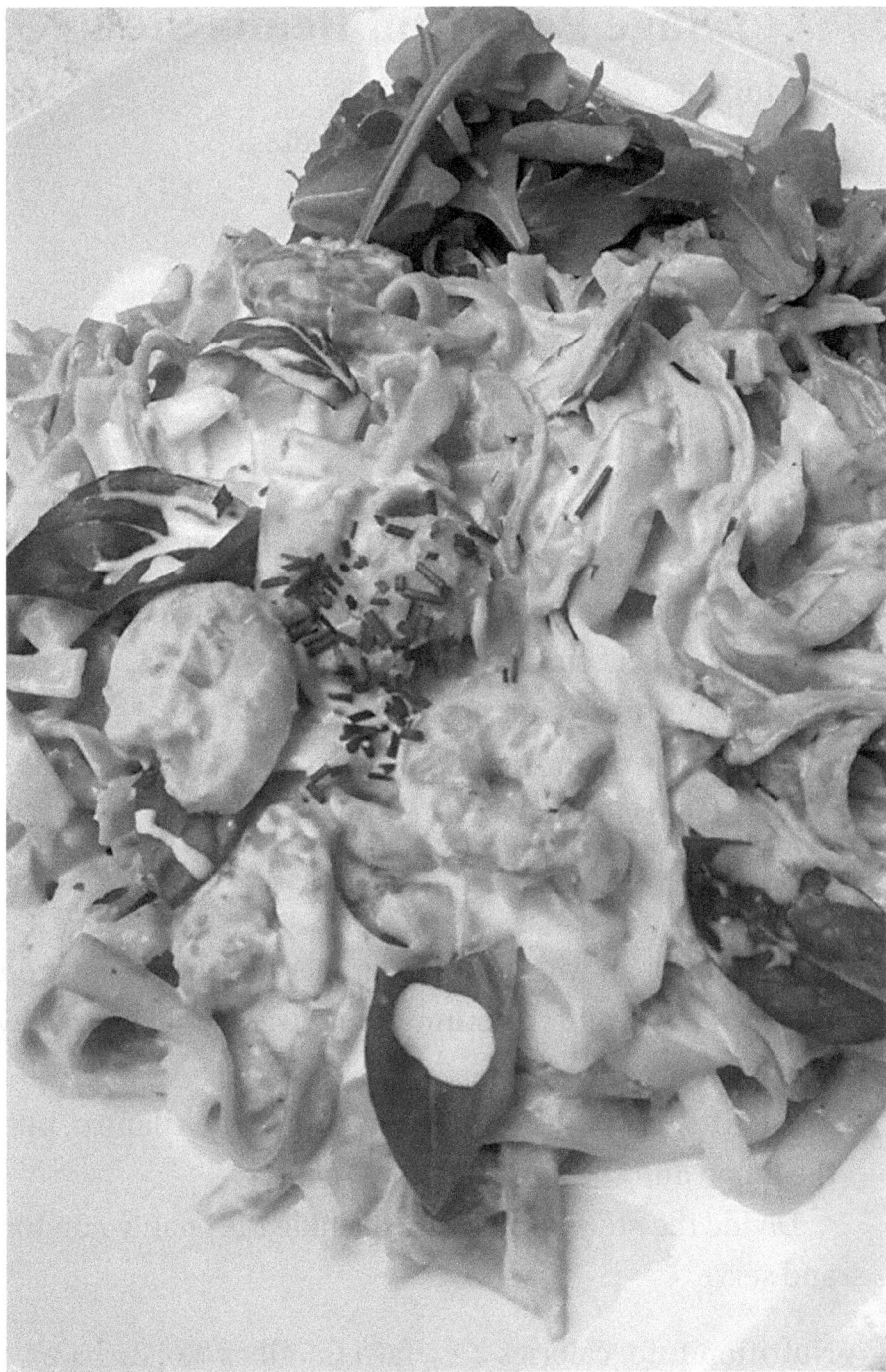

Sage Pork And Beans Stew

Servings: 4

Cooking Time: 4 Hours And 10 Minutes

Ingredients:

- 2 pounds pork stew meat, cubed
- 2 tablespoons olive oil
- 1 sweet onion, chopped
- 1 red bell pepper, chopped
- 3 garlic cloves, minced
- 2 teaspoons sage, dried
- 4 ounces canned white beans, drained
- 1 cup beef stock
- 2 zucchinis, chopped
- 2 tablespoons tomato paste
- 1 tablespoon cilantro, chopped

Directions:

1. Heat up a pan with the oil over medium-high heat, add the meat, brown for 10 minutes and transfer to your slow cooker.

2. Add the rest of the ingredients except the cilantro, put the lid on and cook on High for 4 hours.

3. Divide the stew into bowls, sprinkle the cilantro on top and serve.

Nutrition Info: calories 423, fat 15.4, fiber 9.6, carbs 27.4, protein 43

Broccoli Pesto Spaghetti

Servings: 4
Cooking Time: 35 Minutes

Ingredients:

- 8 oz. spaghetti
- 1 pound broccoli, cut into florets
- 2 tablespoons olive oil
- 4 garlic cloves, chopped
- 4 basil leaves
- 2 tablespoons blanched almonds
- 1 lemon, juiced
- Salt and pepper to taste

Directions:
1. For the pesto, combine the broccoli, oil, garlic, basil, lemon juice and almonds in a blender and pulse until well mixed and smooth.
2. Cook the spaghetti in a large pot of salty water for 8 minutes or until al dente. Drain well.
3. Mix the warm spaghetti with the broccoli pesto and serve right away.

Nutrition Info: Per Serving:Calories:284 Fat:10.2g
Protein:10.4g Carbohydrates:40.2g

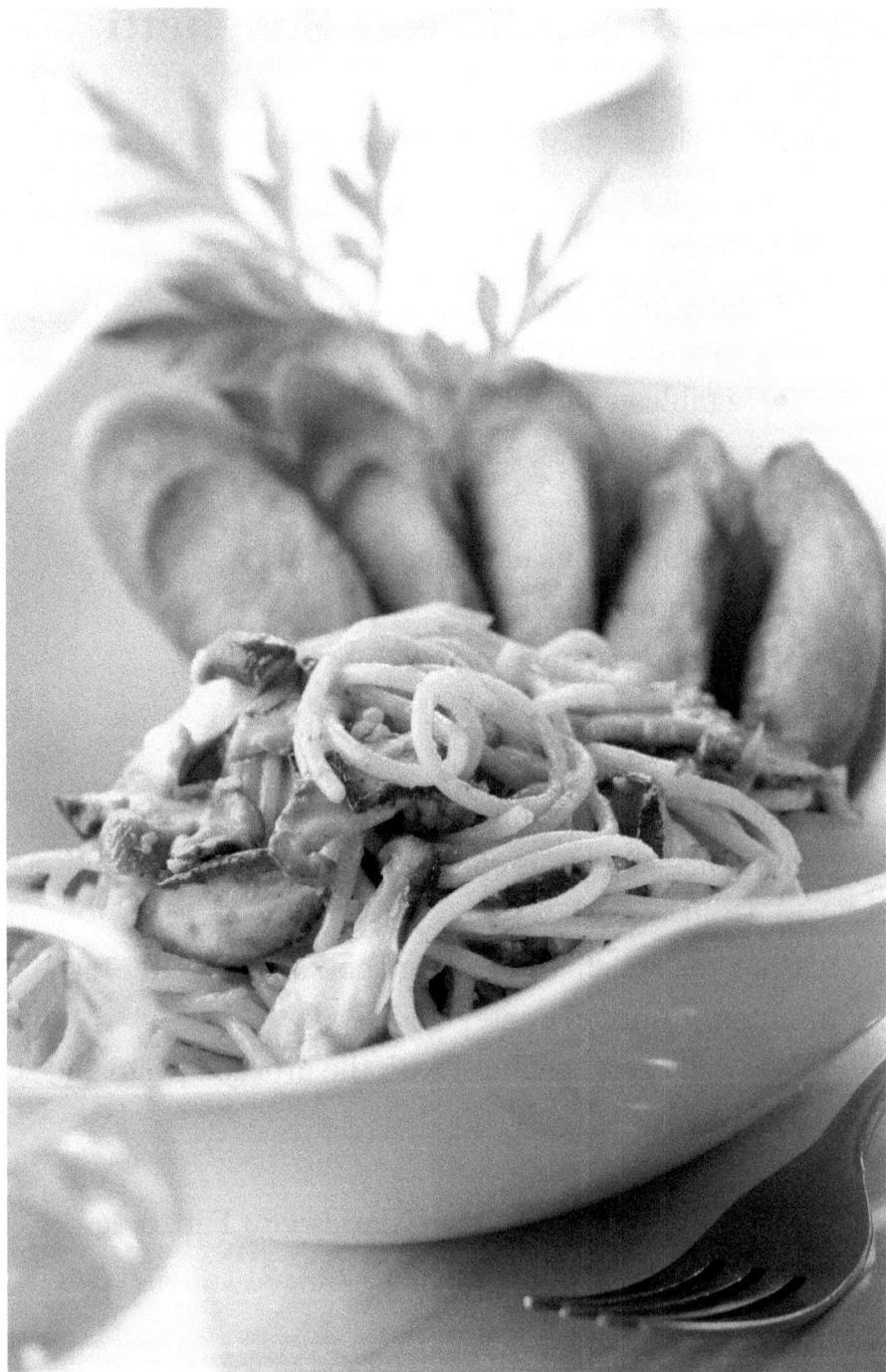

Chorizo Stuffed Chicken Breasts

Servings: 4

Cooking Time: 1 ¼ Hours

Ingredients:

- 4 chicken breasts
- 2 chorizo links, diced
- 4 oz. mozzarella, shredded
- 3 tablespoons olive oil
- 1 shallot, chopped
- 2 garlic cloves, minced
- 1 can diced tomatoes
- ½ cup dry white wine
- ½ cup vegetable stock
- Salt and pepper to taste

Directions:

1. Mix the chorizo and mozzarella in a bowl.

2. Cut a small pocket into each chicken breast and stuff it with the chorizo. 3. Season the chicken with salt and pepper.

4. Heat the oil in a skillet and add the chicken.

5. Cook on each side for 5 minutes or until golden brown.

6. Add the shallot, garlic and tomatoes, as well as wine, stock, salt and pepper.

7. Cook on low heat for 40 minutes.

8. Serve the chicken and the sauce warm.

Nutrition Info: Per Serving:Calories:435 Fat:30.8g Protein:30.2g Carbohydrates:4.2g

Grilled Mediterranean-style Chicken Kebabs

Servings: 10

Cooking Time: 10-15 Minutes

Ingredients:

- 3 chicken filets, diced in 1-inch cubes
- 2 green bell peppers
- 2 red bell peppers
- 1 red onion
- 2 teaspoon black pepper (freshly ground), divided
- 2 teaspoon paprika, divided
- 2 teaspoon thyme, divided
- 2/3 cup extra virgin olive oil, divided
- 4 teaspoon oregano, divided
- 4 teaspoon of salt, divided
- 6 cloves of garlic (minced), divided
- Juice of 1 lemon, divided

Directions:

1. Mix 1/2 amount of all the marinade ingredients in a small bowl, place the chicken in a Ziploc bag and add the marinade. Refrigerate for at least 30 minutes to marinate

2. Mix the remaining 1/2 amount of the marinade ingredients in the same bowl. Pour in the Ziploc bag and add the vegetables. Refrigerate for at least 30 minutes to marinate.

3. When marinated, thread the chicken, the peppers, and the onions into skewers, about 5 to 6 pieces chicken with a combination of onion and peppers between each chicken cubes.

4. Heat an indoor or outdoor grill pan over medium high heat. Lightly oil the grates. Grill the chicken for about 5 minutes per side, or until the center of the cubes are no longer pink.

5. Serve with favorite Mediterranean side dish, salad, or baked potato slices or fries.

Nutrition Info:Per Serving:150 cal., 15 g total fat (2 g sat fat), 0 mg chol., 950 mg sodium, 150 mg potassium, 6 g carb., 2 g fiber, 2 g sugar, and <1 g protein.

Sumac Salmon And Grapefruit

Servings: 4

Cooking Time: 5 Minutes

Ingredients:
- 1 cup parsley leaves, flat-leaf
- 1 teaspoon ground cumin
- 1/4 cup (60ml) olive oil, plus more to brush
- 2 oranges, peeled, segmented
- 2 pink grapefruits, peeled, segmented
- 2 tablespoons sumac
- 4 pieces (180 g each) salmon fillets, skinless, pin-boned
- Juice of 1/2 lemon, and wedges to serve

Directions:

1. In a mixing bowl, combine the sumac and the cumin.

2. Brush the fillets with the olive oil; season with the sumac mixture.

3. In a large frying pan, heat 1 tablespoon olive oil over medium heat. Add the fish fillets; cook for about 2 minutes per side, or until charred on the outside and almost cooked through, but still pink in the middle. Transfer to a plate and loosely cover with foil.

4. Meanwhile, whisk the remaining 2 tablespoons of olive oil and lemon juice; season. Add the fruits and the parsley, toss to coat.

5. Serve the fish fillets with the salad and wedges of lemon.

Nutrition Info:Per Serving:567.9 Cal, 34 g total fat (7 g sat. fat), 16 g carb., 7 g fiber, 47 g protein, and 95.39 mg sodium.

Bean Patties With And Salsa Avocado

Servings: 4

Cooking Time: 10 Minutes

Ingredients:

- 60 g mixed salad leaves, washed, dried
- 5 pieces 13-cm round pocket bread (whole wheat pita bread)
- 1/4 cup chopped fresh coriander
- 1 small red onion, finely chopped
- 1 egg white
- 1 container (170 g) chunky tomato salsa dip
- 1 can (750 g) red kidney beans, rinsed, drained
- 1 avocado, halved, seed removed, peeled, sliced lengthways
- 1 1/2 tablespoons olive oil

Directions:

1. Tear 1 round of pita into pieces; place in the bowl of the food processor and process until breadcrumb-like in texture. Transfer into a medium-sized bowl; set aside.

2. Reserve 185 g (or 1 cup) of the beans; place the remaining beans into the bowl of a food processor. In short bursts, process until roughly mashed.

3. Transfer into a bowl. Add the coriander, onion, reserved beans, egg white, and the pita crumbs; stir well until

combined. With damp hands, divide the mixture into 4 portions, and shape into 8-cm thick and 8-cm wide diameter.

4. In a large nonstick frying pan, heat the oil over medium heat. Add the patties; cook for 4 minutes per side or until golden brown and the patties are heated through.

5. Meanwhile, preheat grill to medium-high. Grill the remaining pita under the preheated grill for about 1 to 2 minutes per side or until toasted.

6. Place the toasted pita into serving plates, top with the mixed salad, the slices of avocado, the bean patties, and the salsa; serve immediately.

Nutrition Info:Per Serving:549 cal., 22 g fat (4 g sat fat), 62 g carb., 8 g sugar, 18 g protein, and 964.9 mg sodium.

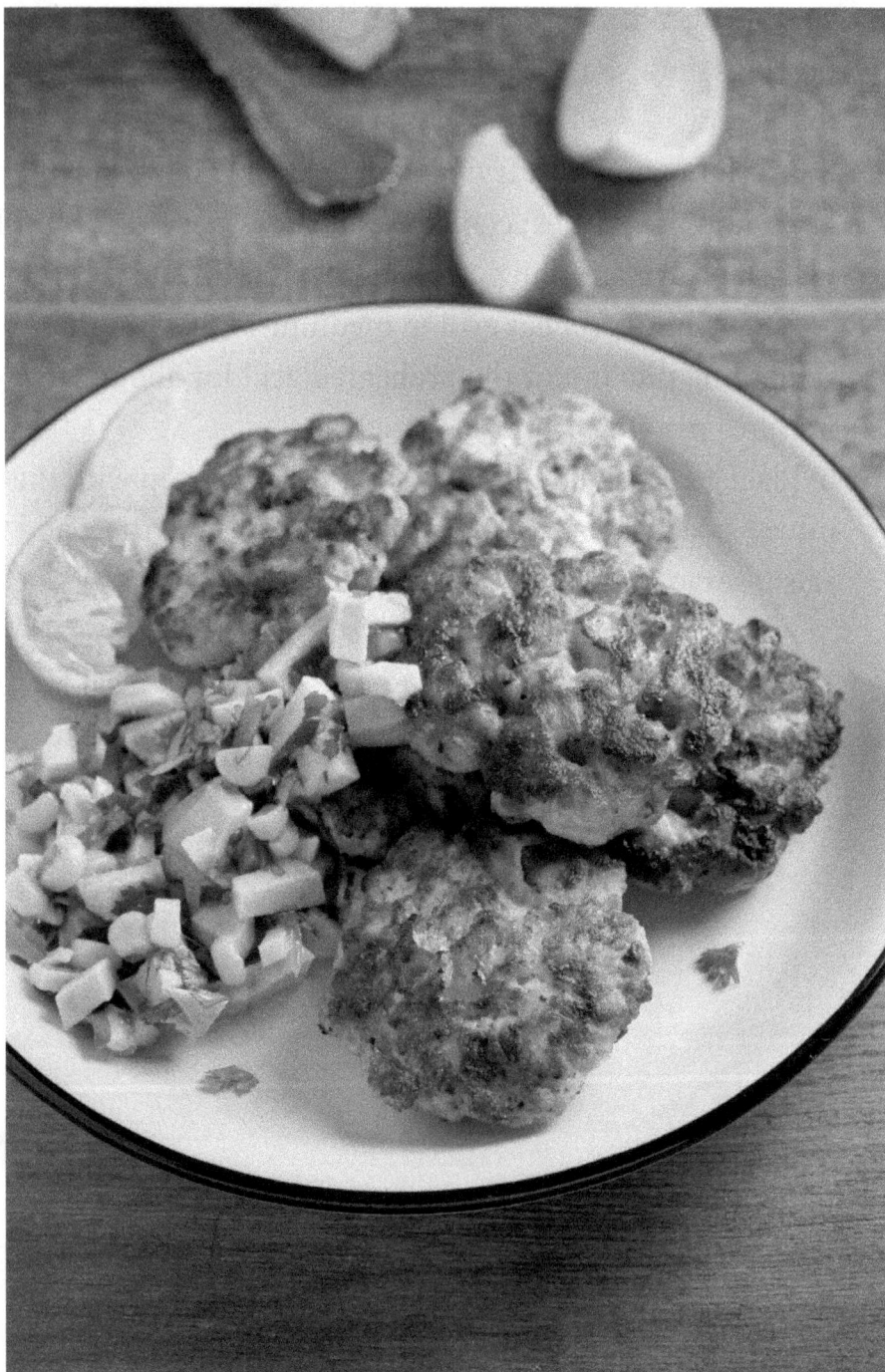

Raisin Stuffed Lamb

Servings: 10
Cooking Time: 2 ½ Hours

Ingredients:
- 4 pounds lamb shoulder
- 1 teaspoon garlic powder
- 1 teaspoon onion powder
- 1 teaspoon chili powder
- Salt and pepper to taste
- 1 cup golden raisins
- 2 red apples, cored and diced
- 1 teaspoon mustard powder
- 1 teaspoon cumin powder
- 2 tablespoons pine nuts
- 1 cup dry white wine

Directions:
1. Season the lamb with garlic powder, onion powder, chili, salt and pepper.
2. Cut a pocket into the lamb.
3. Mix the raisins, red apples, mustard, cumin and pine nuts and stuff the mixture into the lamb.
4. Place the lamb in a deep dish baking pan and cover with aluminum foil.
5. Cook in the preheated oven at 330F for 2 hours.

6. Serve the lamb warm and fresh.

Nutrition Info: Per Serving:Calories:436 Fat:14.8g Protein:52.0g Carbohydrates:18.1g

Spinach Orzo Stew

Servings: 8
Cooking Time: 1 Hour

Ingredients:

- 3 tablespoons olive oil
- 1 sweet onion, chopped
- 2 garlic cloves, minced
- 1 celery stalk, diced
- 2 carrots, diced
- 1 cup orzo, rinsed
- 2 cups vegetable stock
- Salt and pepper to taste
- 4 cups baby spinach
- 1 tablespoon lemon juice

Directions:
1. Heat the oil in a skillet and stir in the onion, garlic, celery and carrots. Cook for 2 minutes until softened then add the orzo.
2. Cook for another 5 minutes then pour in the stock.
3. Add the salt and pepper and cook on low heat for 20 minutes. 4. Add the spinach and lemon juice and cook for another 5 minutes. 5. Serve the stew warm and fresh.

Nutrition Info: Per Serving:Calories:143 Fat:5.8g
Protein:3.5g Carbohydrates:19.8g

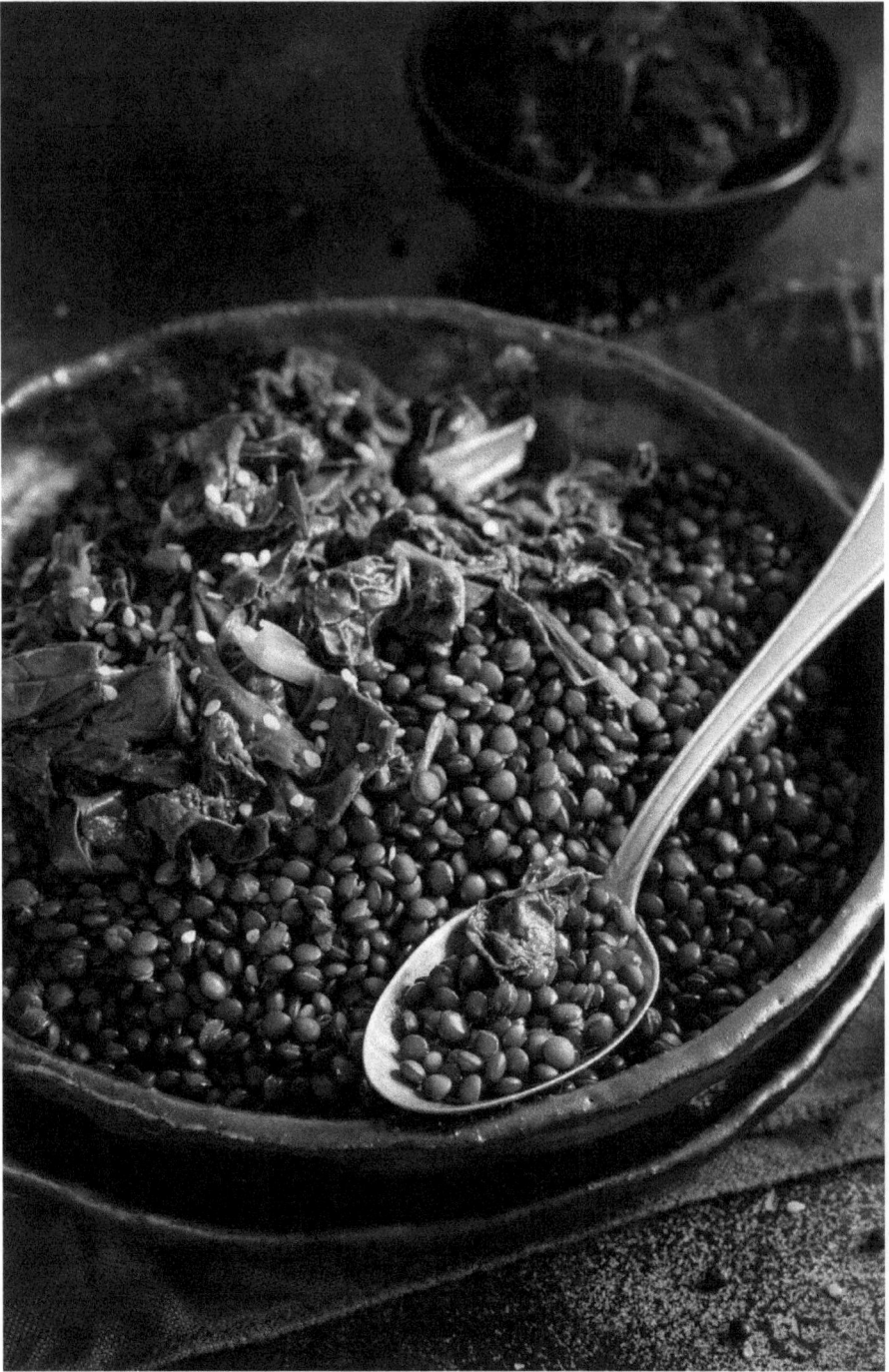

Grapes, Cucumbers And Almonds Soup

Servings: 4
Cooking Time: 0 Minutes

Ingredients:
- ¼ cup almonds, chopped and toasted
- 3 cucumbers, peeled and chopped
- 3 garlic cloves, minced
- ½ cup warm water
- 6 scallions, sliced
- ¼ cup white wine vinegar
- 3 tablespoons olive oil
- Salt and white pepper to the taste
- 1 teaspoon lemon juice
- ½ cup green grapes, halved

Directions:
1. In your blender, combine the almonds with the cucumbers and the rest of the ingredients except the grapes and lemon juice, pulse well and divide into bowls.
2. Top each serving with the lemon juice and grapes and serve cold.

Nutrition Info: calories 200, fat 5.4, fiber 2.4, carbs 7.6, protein 3.3

Nutmeg Beef Soup

Servings: 8

Cooking Time: 30 Minutes

Ingredients:
- 1 yellow onion, chopped
- 1 tablespoon olive oil
- 1 garlic clove, minced
- 1 pound beef meat, ground
- 1 pound eggplant, chopped
- ¾ cup carrots, chopped
- Salt and black pepper to the taste
- 30 ounces canned tomatoes, drained and chopped
- 1 quart beef stock
- ½ teaspoon nutmeg, ground
- 2 teaspoons parsley, chopped

Directions:

1. Heat up a pot with the oil over medium heat, add the meat, onion and the garlic and brown for 5 minutes.

2. Add the rest of the ingredients except the parsley, bring to a boil and cook over medium heat for 25 minutes.

3. Add the parsley, divide the soup into bowls and serve.

Nutrition Info: calories 232, fat 5.4, fiber 7.6, carbs 20.1, protein 6.5

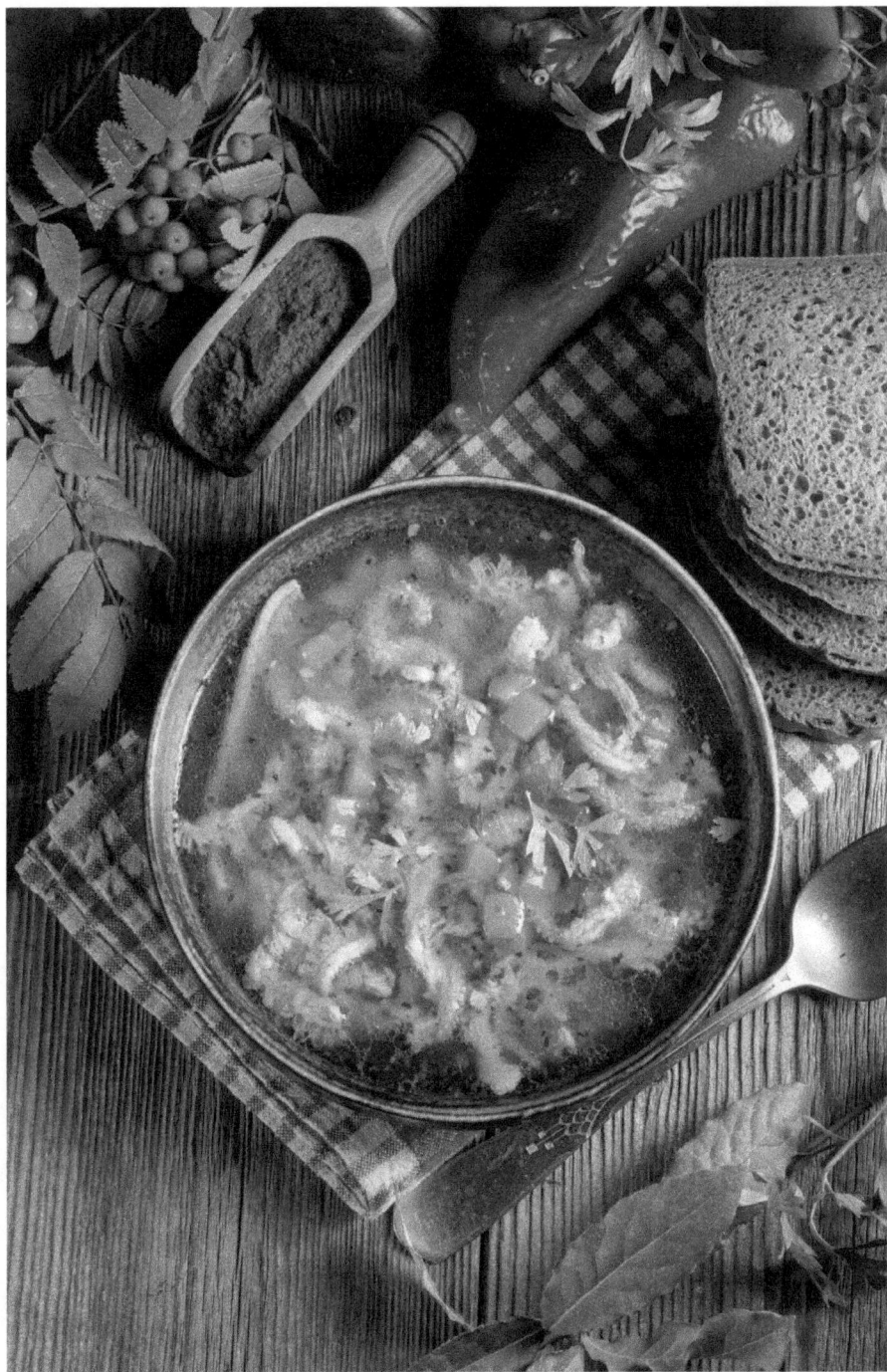

Parsnip Chickpea Veal Stew

Servings: 10

Cooking Time: 2 Hours

Ingredients:

- 2 pounds veal meat, cubed
- 3 tablespoons olive oil
- 2 shallots, chopped
- 4 garlic cloves, chopped
- 2 red bell peppers, cored and sliced
- 2 yellow bell peppers, cored and sliced
- 4 parsnips, peeled and sliced
- 2 carrots, sliced
- 1 can diced tomatoes
- 1 ½ cups beef stock
- 1 bay leaf
- 1 rosemary spring
- 1 oregano spring
- 1 can chickpeas, drained
- Salt and pepper to taste

Directions:

1. Heat the oil in a heavy saucepan and stir in the veal. Cook for 5 minutes until slightly browned.

2. Add the shallots, garlic, bell peppers, parsnips and carrots.

3. Cook for another 5 minutes then stir in the rest of the ingredients.

4. Season with salt and pepper and cook for 1 ½ hours on low heat. 5. Serve the stew warm and fresh.

Nutrition Info: Per Serving:Calories:332 Fat:12.7g Protein:27.8g Carbohydrates:26.9g

Tuna And Couscous

Servings: 4
Cooking Time: 0 Minutes

Ingredients:
- 1 cup chicken stock
- 1 and ¼ cups couscous
- A pinch of salt and black pepper
- 10 ounces canned tuna, drained and flaked
- 1 pint cherry tomatoes, halved
- ½ cup pepperoncini, sliced
- 1/3 cup parsley, chopped
- 1 tablespoon olive oil
- ¼ cup capers, drained
- Juice of ½ lemon

Directions:
1. Put the stock in a pan, bring to a boil over medium-high heat, add the couscous, stir, take off the heat, cover, leave aside for 10 minutes, fluff with a fork and transfer to a bowl.
2. Add the tuna and the rest of the ingredients, toss and serve for lunch right away.

Nutrition Info: calories 253, fat 11.5, fiber 3.4, carbs 16.5, protein 23.2

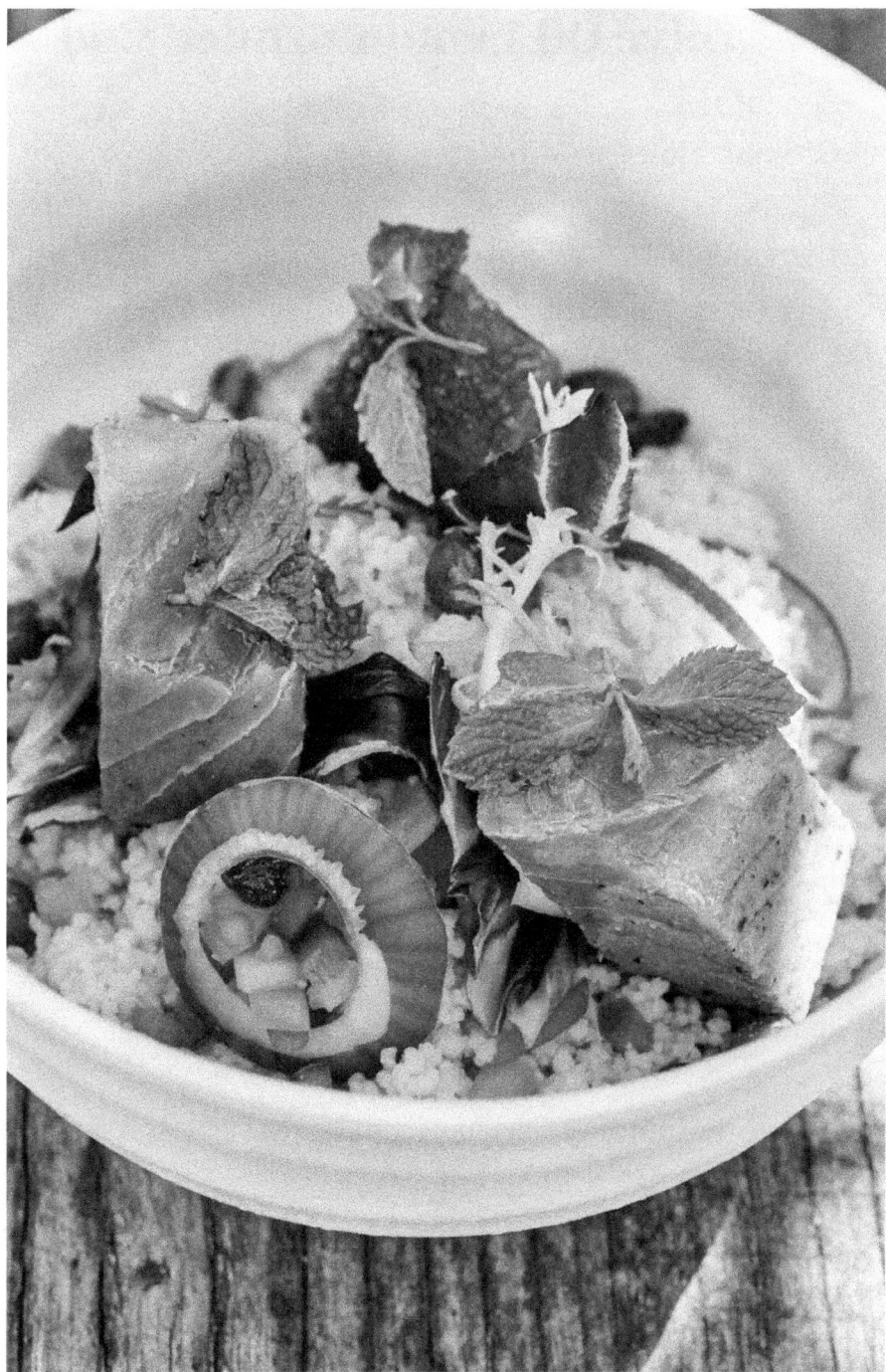

Olive Oil Lemon Broiled Cod

Servings: 4

Cooking Time: 35 Minutes

Ingredients:

- 4 cod fillets
- 1 teaspoon dried marjoram
- 4 tablespoons olive oil
- 1 lemon, juiced
- 1 thyme spring
- Salt and pepper to taste

Directions:

1. Season the cod with salt, pepper and marjoram.
2. Heat the oil in a large skillet and place the cod in the hot oil. 3. Fry on medium heat on both sides until golden brown then add the lemon juice.
4. Place the thyme sprig on top and cover with a lid.
5. Cook for 5 more minutes then remove from heat.
6. Serve the cod and sauce fresh.

Nutrition Info: Per Serving:Calories:304 Fat:15.5g Protein:40.0g Carbohydrates:0.1g

Notes